Lacanian Psychoanalysis and American Literature

Lacanian Psychoanalysis and American Literature considers the psychoanalytic applications of three classic works of nineteenth-century literature, applying Lacanian concepts throughout.

Moncayo imports the dynamisms and texture of three English and American stories with the aim of developing psychoanalytic theory, rather than simply confirming or applying previously adopted psychoanalytic concepts and theory. The author begins with *The Purloined Letter* by Edgar Allan Poe, assessing the differences between Derrida's and Lacan's analysis of this famous story. The book then considers *The Turn of the Screw* by Henry James, using James' text for an in-depth analysis of Lacan's Seminar on the *Logic of the Fantasy*, and *Wuthering Heights* by Emily Brontë, considering "passage à l'acte", and the *objet a* as the Wind and Heart of the Signifier. The authors use Lacan's later theories to cast a new interpretative light on the stories, much as Lacan himself did with the work of James Joyce.

Lacanian Psychoanalysis and American Literature will be of interest to academics and scholars of literary studies, psychoanalytic and Lacanian studies, and Philosophy.

Raul Moncayo, PhD, is a supervising analyst and past founding member and former president of the Lacanian School of Psychoanalysis, USA. He is the author of seven books on Lacanian Psychoanalysis. Together with Yang Yu and Hong Zhou, he founded the Beijing Center for Freudian and Lacanian Psychoanalysis and Research to transmit a Lacanian psychoanalysis with an ongoing, active engagement with Chinese culture. In 2019, he founded the Blue Mountain Zen Center of El Cerrito, California.

Lacanian Psychoanalysis and American Literature

Metaphoric Truth, Imaginary Fiction, Letter Jouissance, and Nomination

Raul Moncayo

Routledge
Taylor & Francis Group
LONDON AND NEW YORK

Designed cover image: Getty | themacx

First published 2024
by Routledge
4 Park Square, Milton Park, Abingdon, Oxon OX14 4RN

and by Routledge
605 Third Avenue, New York, NY 10158

Routledge is an imprint of the Taylor & Francis Group, an informa business

British Library Cataloguing-in-Publication Data
A catalogue record for this book is available from the British Library

ISBN: 9781032543765 (hbk)
ISBN: 9781032543758 (pbk)
ISBN: 9781003424574 (ebk)

DOI: 10.4324/9781003424574

Typeset in Times New Roman
by codeMantra

Contents

Acknowledgments

This book would not have happened if it were not for the invitation of my student Yang Yu from Beijing Normal University. The talks were given over a period of a month and Professor Yu contributed to their preparation. I am especially indebted to her for her general editing and her contributions to the last chapter, where she developed several of Lacan's formulas for metaphor and metonymy.

Finally, this book is also dedicated to my British primary school English teacher who helped me discover that English was my mother tongue.

Chapter 1

Introduction

The Contemporary State of North American Literature

For some literary scholars, contemporary literary studies may contain too much discussion of non-literary matters, and too much reading of difficult psychoanalytical and philosophical texts, for example. From this perspective, literary studies should be more like linguistics, and be focused on the formal aspects of literary productions. Literary theory should be focused on questions such as, "What is the formal structure of the language in a text in terms of grammar rules, syntax, and different figures and forms of language?" However, a poem or novel that does not contain high or low points of human experience could hardly formally qualify as Literature. Therefore, regardless of methodology, literary criticism cannot ignore the dimension of human experience in a literary work.

Both Literature and Psychoanalysis share an interest in serving as a means to reveal the linguistic and psychical patterning available within the structure of the language that we use and that structures our lives. In this sense, truth is half-fiction, as Lacan said, or we could say that truth is half revealed in literary fiction. In "A Room of One's Own", Virginia Woolf also expresses a similar idea, "Fiction here is likely to contain more truth than fact" (2). The so-called literary fiction becomes something more than fiction, and at the same time there is something fictional in objective representational truth insofar as it represents an approximation to the absolute reality of things in themselves.

At the other end, there are those who think that literature's main function is to describe human experience in meaningful ways without relying on speculative theory. A psychoanalytic reading of narrative histories is somewhere in between and uses both experience and underlying psychical, logical, and linguistic structures to elucidate a text. The analysis of form in language says something about human desire that, in the case of literature, is also pleasant for the reader. The fact that literature is of interest to human beings, or is an indispensable aspect of human activity, is intrinsically or structurally related to the act of reading as a form of jouissance or satisfaction. In line with this, for many critics a story is "Freudian" if it arouses certain subjective responses in the reader.

I find a dichotomy between the formal analysis of a text or narrative and a theoretical and an experiential approach to the same. The good news is that psychoanalysis as a discourse includes all three. Psychoanalysis is a discourse, a theory,

DOI: 10.4324/9781003424574-1

and a clinical or analytical practice. The story is never divorced from social and normative narratives and yet psychoanalytic theory is more than this since it has a theory about the relations among stories, unconscious signifying chains, symptoms, and various forms of affect and jouissance. The stories are the ideologies, while the signifying chain represents the logic of fantasy embedded within a text. As Fredric Jameson insists, literary creation is always structurally unconscious, while the signifying chain represents the logic of fantasy embedded within a text.

In contrast to Jameson or Eagleton I do not consider psychoanalysis as an ideological form of discourse. Ideologies, and mythologies, as complete discourses are in the narrative level of discourse and the graph of desire. Instead, psychoanalytic discourse, as an incomplete and consistent science, organizes its theory and practice around an unconscious signifying chain that links narrative discourse and ideology to the symptom. Ideology is part of the problem, rather than the solution for the symptom. The solution to the problem of the symptom and human suffering lies in the unconscious signifying chain rather than ideology.

But what are the correspondences between the formal analysis of literary texts from contemporary literary and theoretical perspectives, and the way that theory and practice function within psychoanalysis as a science and treatment method?

First, there is the theory of narrative (narratology) that has been an active branch of literary theory. Literary studies rely on theories of narrative structure: for example, what events are described in a plot, what are the elements of a plot or a story, what discourse is being presented, and/or what narrative techniques are being used?

When the question of discourse or cultural critique (of colonialism in postcolonial theory, for example) is introduced into literary analysis, the question of theory becomes inevitable. However, theory or conceptual thought in psychoanalysis is not without evidence since the theory is inseparable from its practice. When applied to literary analysis the evidence is not in the biography of the author, however relevant this may be, since all we have is a text, no more, no less. There is no use in "speculating" about what elements of the plot represented this or that in the life of the author. In literature we find similar voices from Oscar Wilde and one of his characters when they say, "To reveal art and conceal the artist is art's aim" (3) and

> An artist should create beautiful things but should put nothing of his own life into them. We live in an age when people treat art as if it were meant to be a form of autobiography. We have lost the abstract sense of beauty.
>
> (14)

Psychoanalysis uses theory derived from such varied fields as anthropology, literature, sociology, including mathematics and topology in the case of Lacan. This is not unlike the theory used in literary studies that includes works of art history, film studies, linguistics, etc. Psychoanalysis, as distinct from literary analysis, stops short of being interdisciplinary in the sense that the theory, which could contain elements from other fields, nevertheless always focuses on the speech-acts and events of the analysand.

Critique is also common to literary studies and psychoanalysis. Writing, as well as free association, is a form of reconciling the contradictions in society and the subject that otherwise can lead to misunderstanding or miscommunication in ordinary social speech. Critique also involves a reflection and a check on the categories and assumptions used in speech. Ezra Pound categorized "The Turn of the Screw", for example, as a literary protest "against all the sordid petty personal crushing oppression, the domination of modern life". James' work has already been interpreted as hovering over between being a psychological or psychical modern novel describing the psychical life of twentieth-century characters (the governess's ghosts are her own personal mental hallucinations), at the turn of the century, and his own brother's interest in the "psychical" that refers to the belief in the afterlife, death, seances, and invoking the ghosts that haunt the living.

With respect to the question of experience and whether there is an objective reality outside language or a text, these two are not the same thing. Objective reality could refer not to visual images that are always deceptive, but rather to mathematical structure, something that otherwise is entirely plausible. In addition, outside the text or language refers to the question of the Real and jouissance, and the subjective experience involved in both writing and reading. Different genres of writing afford different forms of jouissance and respond to different forms of interest. With the speech of the analysand in analysis the question of jouissance between reader and writer, analyst and analysand, is always present.

Nevertheless, in the case of Lacan the question of jouissance still has a logical and topological structure and is not simply a form of emotional irrationality or romanticism without structure. In addition, although psychoanalysis uses the storytelling or narrative aspect of speech, it considers this level of speech not its fundamental object of investigation. Psychoanalysis is concerned with the unconscious signifying chain as its topological substratum and what jouissance is invoked or weaved for the reader by the localized brilliance of a necklace of metaphors shining like bright pearls.

The question of the relative importance of structure or signification versus jouissance in a text is also implicated in the aesthetic understanding of a text as a work of art. How much is a text a question of forces, magnitudes, and artistic beauty, versus a question of signifiers, and conceptual or logical structure. In addition, in Literature, not only grammatical structure but also artistic style, or the way an author writes and/or tells a story, is important. Artistic style is what distinguishes one author from another, and creates a unique voice that readers want to hear.

In Lacanian analysis, style is also important for detecting the uniqueness of an author or a text. But style is more than simply an artistic feature. In the *Ecrits*, Lacan says that readers will know about his style by reading his text on "The Purloined Letter". "My style" here is a pun referring to both Lacan's style and Lacan's psychoanalytic definition of style. An easy entry into style is through understanding that the destination of the letter is always to be lost. This is how we understand how truth inhabits fiction. Truth inhabits fiction as causality in the form a gap, or something missing within the structure of the signifier. The letter designates propositional truth, but this truth can never fully manifest itself without the subject's own fictional misrecognition of his/her fate, and the narcissistic rationalization of this fate in his/her memory.

Lacan's writing style is unique, ornamented, and highly metaphorical. In the *Ecrits*, he uses this style to talk about style itself. Some readers take *Ecrits*' difficult writing style as Lacan's symptom or problem in writing. At best, Lacan's writing has been described or critiqued as being abstruse, obtuse, and cryptic, while, at worst, his writing has been parodied or ridiculed as incoherent, chaotic, and confused. Lacan's style is cryptic or obtuse because, like meaning, the letter and its destiny and destination is always to be lost, to be missing, and in absentia. Literature is fiction because its truth is always missing or concealed and needs to be "read" and deciphered by the reader. Truth can never fully manifest itself without the subject's own fictional misrecognition of their fate, his/her identification with their "semblable", and secondarily without narcissistically conveniently rationalizing this fate in their memory. Self-reference, when the self in self-reference refers to the ego, is always highly problematical. When subjects lose themselves in the signifier, the reference is always metaphorical.

Yes, Lacan's style is his symptom, but, more than that, the symptom also shows Lacan's distinct approach to psychoanalysis and writing. In this sense, his style is also his sinthome. "The style is the man himself". The symptom represents the person, while the singularity is in the person. The sinthome is the person in himself/herself, and beyond themselves. In literature, the example for a person of style is Oscar Wilde, who not only spoke and wrote about style, but also lived "in style".

In addition, the question of a person's style does not point to self-love and a person's narcissistic or histrionic "flair", as Lacan's style has sometimes been ridiculed. Like the formal signifier, style represents the subject, and leads away from the ego individual as the reference point. The perception of style is a question of style posed to the Other, and where the answer comes back to the subject in inverted form. The meaning of the statement "The man is the style" is heard backward. Paradoxically, or ironically, although man appears to be focus, the actual reference is the style rather than the person.

Art, beauty, and style, all refer to questions of love and desire more than technical knowledge, although not exclusively. Literary theorists and psychoanalysts in general ask questions about both: what are the links among desire, stories, psychical structure, and formal knowledge about language?

> Since the point is to take desire, and since it can only be taken literally [*a la lettre*], since it is the letter's snare that determines, nay overdetermines, its place as a heavenly bird, how can we fail to require the bird catcher to first be a man of letters?
>
> (*Ecrits*, 2006, p. 536)

Desire cannot be found in ordinary speech acts. Desire is weaved at the letter level, the same level as the construction of the word itself. Lacan creatively uses the expression "man of letters" in the sense that the literary person, the writer, who gets us in contact with jouissance because jouissance structurally belongs to the letter. So, a jouissance of words or of the signifier could be only explained by the letter. For the Lacan of the Purloined Letter period, the real is the syntax underlying automaton, which is the ultimate reason of symbolic determination and yet cannot be fully symbolized in speech. For the later Lacan, it is the creative use of the letter within the Real unconscious (lalangue, or the language of the One) that generates jouissance.

The letter's snare overdetermines the apparent irrationality of desire, or its place as a bird of paradise, as Lacan says, and this is suggestive of satisfaction but also of suffering and loss. Loss of the beloved, or loss of love, is linked to how the letter comes to represent a hole in "the ardent place of the heart".

The poetic function of language as conceived by Roman Jakobson is not different from how language works within linguistic and unconscious mental structure as "lalangue" or the language of what the later Lacan calls the Real unconscious. In the Real unconscious links and associations are established through homophony, phonemes, and the sounds of the letters in language. Jakobson gives the example of a political slogan from the American presidential campaign of Dwight D. ("Ike") Eisenhower: "I like Ike". Through the homophonic link, the necessity of liking or the desire for Ike seems inscribed in the very structure of the language. As the phoneme was the basic unit of analysis for understanding the signifier and the repressed unconscious in the middle period of his work, homophony between phonemes becomes the basic unit of analysis for the Real unconscious of Lacan's later work.

The poetic function of language, as Lacan argues, and as demonstrated in this book, is also related to the way that metaphor is linked to the production of the subject and the cancellation of the imaginary ego. In a sense, psychoanalysis is both a science and a poetic art. The voice of a text is not the imaginary ego, but rather the I of the signifier that speaks for what otherwise would be an imaginary ego. The ego thinks that language advances the purposes and aims of the ego, while in actuality it is the pure signifier that advances and realizes the subject.

Recent theorists, such as Kristeva, have argued for intertextuality or for the notion that works are made out of other works that they take up, repeat, challenge, and transform. The notion of two or more texts and languages interacting is also found in psychical structure. The two forms of language interact with two modalities of mental structure: Psyche and Mind, desire and defense. There are the laws of language, the language of the code and censorship, and then there is the language of desire and jouissance as its structural underside. Cs. Pcs. language interacts with the language of the unconscious, with sometimes one (Cs. Pcs.) representing the language of defense, and the other, the language of desire and jouissance, while at other times, the perspectives, or the alignment between the two languages and the two aspect of psyche and mind are reversed. Sometimes the language of desire becomes a language of defense against jouissance so that desire can be reached through “the inverted ladder of the law”.

This is a topological description of psychical reality. In speech there are always modalities and transformations acting upon letters, defenses, desires, and jouissance. So, the human Mind is always both logical and poetical, objective/abstract, and subjective. That is why dyadic intersubjectivity cannot escape an imaginary fate, while the dialectical movements of signifiers are always beyond dualism, and sometimes beyond the Symbolic when the signified is located within a bodily experience of jouissance and the register of the Real.

Finally, the book is organized in a way that leads and culminates with the last chapter functioning as a conclusion and opening new avenues for research on metaphor and its function for psychoanalysis in its relations with Tyche as a principle of “undetermination”. The theses and formulas for metaphor were built with and developed with the help of Chinese English professor Yu Yang.

Reference

Lacan, J. (2006). Ecrits. New York: Norton & Norton

Chapter 2

Literary Gems and the Psychical Logic of the Text

Truth is half-fiction, or truth has the structure of fiction, as Lacan said, or, for purposes of this book, we will say that truth is half revealed in literary fiction. Representational truth is half-fiction because the entire truth cannot be said in language. Language cannot say the Truth about truth. The fictional side of truth also represents the "disputational" aspect of truth where different actors may hold different and opposing versions of it.

Azari (2008) mentions that "The frontier between the two fields of literature and psychoanalysis often remains unchecked and unguarded" (p. 93). To this field we would also add philosophy since Derrida was a philosopher more than a literary scholar. For this reason, he criticizes Lacan for lack of formal philosophical rigor. In addition, Derrida also criticizes Lacan for not having enough interest or background in literature. Of course, that there is ample evidence of Lacan's literary interests in his writing, and there are many specialists who also think of Lacan as a literary theorist. For example, Azari argues that "Lacan's interpretation of literature, instead, is a guideline, a street directory that shows us the causes of events and behavior of characters in a text and of the content, messages, structure, plot, rhythm and other fundamental constituents of literature" (p. 93).

Lacan uses riddles and enigmas, respects the literary structure of the text, and traces the itinerary of the Letter. Instead of psychobiography, Lacan had great respect for literary critics who discussed the process and structure of a text in terms of motif, theme, plot, narrative, structure, surface, symbol, and consistency.

Lacan had a wish to leave literature in the domain of riddles and enigmas that he associated to "La Troisieme" or the third jouissance of meaning. "Jouis-Sense" is the third jouissance of hearing the riddles and gaps in meaning, which differs from a "too much" or a proliferation of double Imaginary meaning, and from signification in language according to the logic of the signifier.

Literary scholars can criticize psychoanalysts for dabbling in analytical literary analysis without sufficient background in literature, while psychoanalysts can critique literary scholars and philosophers for dabbling and critiquing psychoanalytic theory without sufficient clinical experience or background in psychoanalysis. Is it true that the literary Lacan is more important than the psychoanalyst for literature and literary theory? It seems this could be the opinion of literary scholars.

DOI: 10.4324/9781003424574-2

We are not sure that psychoanalysts would say that psychoanalytic case examples and theory are more important than reading literature for the formation of analysts. Although this is concretely true, Lacan quoted Freud in saying that literature is a pre-requisite for the training of analysts, and many analysts have enjoyed and learned much about psychoanalysis through reading literature as an artistic fictional record, not unlike many life stories heard in analysis. Perhaps here we should remind ourselves of the obvious fact that Freud in no small measure developed a psychoanalytic theory of mind from reading Oedipus Rex. Through Freud's and Lacan's study of many historical literary figures, literature is weaved into the construction of psychoanalysis and embedded within its structure.

Lacan appears to be less critical of Derrida, or lay analysts, although analysts have not failed to mention that Derrida was not a clinician although he was a philosopher with clinical aspirations. In this regard, the border of psychoanalysis also lies unguarded as Azari says. The study of psychoanalysis in the humanities has led many scholars to dabble into analytical practice without prior clinical, psychological, or psychiatric formation. Although both Freud and Lacan supported the idea of a lay analyst, they both had extensive and varied clinical experience. A partial current situation, where literary scholars may note the alleged clinical failures or poor outcomes of analytic treatment as proof that psychoanalysis is mainly a signifying practice as a form of literary or textual analysis, is echoed in biological psychiatry (for different interests) nowadays that summarily dismisses psychoanalysis as being literary analysis rather than a treatment method.

If for no other reason, the current book is written by a psychoanalyst who is a practitioner-scholar. However, I remained indebted to Professor Yang Yu of Beijing Normal University's English department, who is a scholar and a research analyst. She read and contributed to the book. The psychoanalyst has studied psychoanalysis more than literature, and the reverse is true for the literary scholar. When studying Lacan, one is studying both a literary and a psychoanalytical text. I wanted for Professor Yu to guard the border of literary theory for me.

Lacan did not support applying psychoanalysis to literature because psychoanalysis can only be applied in the clinic. Instead, I follow Lacan in a desire to import some of the dynamisms of the text to develop psychoanalytic theory. Lacan begins with literary references and stylistic effects, and finally moves into the theoretical articulation of the text. We do not seek to prove already established concepts, but to develop them, and create new ones without too much proliferation.

The new is always measured by the topological criteria of the rubber sheet: you can bend it, stretch it, make it change form, and yet the structure is preserved. The entire universe is made up of vibrating strings. Old concepts are replaced by new ones with increased explanatory power, but the structure is preserved.

In the case of Lacanian theory, the Borromean knot increases the explanatory power of psychoanalysis, while at the same time preserving its structure. If psychoanalysts interpret texts to prove established concepts, moreover if they think the text can be reduced to the interpretation, then their judgments on the text are not as important for literature as those of literary critics. The text has to be used for scientific purposes to develop psychoanalysis as a theory and a practice.

Freud's text contained truths as conceptual metaphors not as facts or data. We use metaphor, not metonymy, to develop psychoanalysis as a science, while metonymy is more for the field of literary studies proper as fiction. Freud invented literary metaphors, and for this he was nominated for the Nobel Prize for Literature. But then the question immediately arises whether it is possible to have a metaphor without metonymy?

For human beings, there is always an interaction between metaphor and metonymy, or otherwise there will be no desire. What is possible is to discern whether metaphor has ascendancy over metonymy or metonymy has ascendancy over metaphor, just as the logic of fantasy shows. Literature uses displaced metaphors to reveal the metonymic structure of desire, while psychoanalysis uses conceptual metaphors to handle and reveal the underlying symbolic structure of the fantasy.

In psychoanalysis the distortion of truth is recognized in metonymy. The truth of desire in the imaginary is an untruth for the truth of metaphor, and the truth of desire is an untruth for the truth of metaphor. Imaginary truth is sublated into the truth of metaphor that is more effective than an ideological normative discourse against the untruths of desire that in the end is ideology rather than science.

Logically organized metaphors are more important to understand the human mind, than data or information extracted from numbers that have been artificially produced based on the researcher's own assumptions, and the responses of the research subjects to these assumptions. The signifiers of the subject are not coded, and instead the responses related to the researcher's assumptions are. Psychoanalysis uses the language used by the subject to conduct its investigations. Metaphor is the data that is used to organize the structure of the theory.

Theory is not a climate of opinion, fashion, or hearsay that changes continually after the mores and ideology of the culture. Theory is a progressive series of constructions and amplifications, just like Einstein's theory explains things that Newton's theory did not explain, some things he explains better, but Newton's theory is not invalidated and is a pre-condition of Einstein's theory. We argue something similar with respect to Freud and Lacan, except that there are aspects of Freud's theory that still correct and contribute to Lacanian theory. This is one of our hypotheses. We are not sure the same thing could be said about Einstein and Newton, thus justifying and legitimizing Lacan's cry of a Return to Freud. We follow Lacan in returning to Freud to develop Lacanian theory. However, Freud would be ashamed of Lacan's reduction of psychoanalysis to a literature that can be sold (Rabate, p. 81).

Through a process of induction, literary metaphor and metonymy are transformed into conceptual metaphors. Mental contents (so-called "experiential concretes") such as feelings or thoughts are not inserted into signifying containers (as cognitive linguistics believes) such as letters, words, phrases, sentences because the former are already both, and the latter structure the former. So, what we need are concepts that are conceptual metaphors that are logically and even mathematically organized.

The written symbol in mathematics represents a series of equations and processes that have already been proven and demonstrated. Symbols are used to relate diverse fields of knowledge and mathematics. Mathematical symbols are a web of connections, an intellectual Nexus providing a bridge across subjects and connecting seemingly disparate ideas. Conceptual Metaphors, like Names in language in their singular nominative aspect (Nomination), in this respect, function as a conceptual nexus that stops the sliding of metonymy to give us a singular representation of a topic or subject. Equations are the logical articulation of symbols to represent a hypothesis. The equivalent of a metaphoric symbol as a web of connections in language would be a genealogical tree. Ancestors are equations that have already been proven and that lead to the construction of a new personal equation.

But what are the correspondences between the formal analysis of literary texts and contemporary literary and theoretical perspectives, and the way that theory and practice function within psychoanalysis as a science and treatment method?

First, there is the theory of narrative (narratology) that has been an active branch of literary theory. Literary studies rely on theories of narrative structure: for example, what events are described in a plot, what are the elements of a plot or a story, what discourse is being presented, and/or what narrative techniques are being used?

When the question of discourse or cultural critique (of colonialism in postcolonial theory, for example) is introduced into literary analysis, the question of theory becomes inevitable. However, theory or conceptual thought in psychoanalysis is not without evidence since the theory is inseparable from its practice. When applied to literary analysis the evidence is not in the biography of the author, however relevant this may be, since all we have is a text, no more, no less. There is no use in "speculating" about what elements of the plot represented this or that in the life of the author. In literature we find similar voices in Oscar Wilde and one of his characters when they say, "To reveal art and conceal the artist is art's aim" (3) and

> An artist should create beautiful things but should put nothing of his own life into them. We live in an age when people treat art as if it were meant to be a form of autobiography. We have lost the abstract sense of beauty.
>
> (14)

Lacanian theory breaks away from any thematic analysis of a text or a narrative and foregoes a primary reference or analysis of a story based on the psychobiography, childhood experience, or personality of the author. Although an author may be motivated in their research by personal factors, the structure of a discourse is determined by non-personal symbolic factors. Psychoanalysis focuses on the key signifiers emergent in a subject's speech that represent the unconscious signifying chain rather than the conscious narrative. The narrative of the analysand in analysis is not necessarily interpreted in terms of the social or family history of the conscious subject. The stories that are told and said are analyzed in the logical and emotional terms of the unconscious signifying chain.

More than the conscious family narrative, it is the unconscious signifying chain that manifests the truths of the subject. Similarly, in the analysis of a literary text, the narrative and the plot represent the surface narrative, while the symbolic and psychical structure of human desire embody the intelligibility of the text as a theoretical and scientific discourse. In Lacanian theory the analysis of the symbolic and mental structure of desire within a text occupies the place that psychobiography occupies in Freud's work. Freud interpreted the elements of a story in terms of historical or family childhood events, while Lacan, also following Freud, privileges the unconscious signifying chain to reveal and work through the mental and emotional truths associated with desire.

Psychoanalysis uses theory derived from such varied fields as anthropology, literature, sociology, including mathematics and topology in the case of Lacan. This is not unlike the theory used in literary studies that includes works of art, history, film studies, linguistics, etc. Psychoanalysis, as distinct from literary analysis and other social discourses, stops short of being multidisciplinary in the sense that the theory, which could contain elements from other fields, nevertheless always focuses on the speech-acts and events of the analysand.

Critique is also common to literary studies and psychoanalysis. Writing as well as free association are forms of reconciling the contradictions in society and the subject that otherwise can lead to misunderstanding or miscommunication in ordinary social speech. Critique also involves a reflection and a check on the categories and assumptions used in speech. James' work has already been interpreted as hovering over between being a psychological or psychical modern novel describing the psychical life of twentieth-century characters (the governess's ghosts are her own personal mental hallucinations), at the turn of the century, and his own brother's interest in the "psychical" that in his case referred to a belief in the afterlife, death, seances, and invoking the ghosts that haunt the living.

With respect to the question of experience and whether there is an objective reality outside language or a text, these two are not the same thing. Objective reality could refer not to visual images that are always deceptive, but rather to mathematical structure, something that otherwise is entirely plausible. In addition, outside the text or language refers to the question of the Real and jouissance, and the subjective experience involved in both writing and reading. Different genres of writing afford different forms of jouissance and respond to different forms of interest. With speech and the uttering of phonemes in analysis the question of jouissance between reader and writer, analyst and analysand, is always present.

In the reading of a text, the only interaction is between the text and the subjectivity of the reader. Similar to what happens in analysis, a narrative fiction contains more truth than seen at the narrative level because there is always a beyond that refers to unconscious structure. However, a reader can only reconstruct the beyond the text based on their subjective experiences or on theoretical elaborations. In the experience of analysis, the analyst has to use the analysand's free associative material to reach the unconscious. This is not the same as how a reader could use introspection to elaborate on their subjective responses to a text.

Nevertheless, in the case of Lacan, the question of jouissance still has a logical and topological structure and is not simply a form of emotional irrationality or romanticism without structure. In addition, although psychoanalysis uses the story-telling or narrative aspect of speech, it considers this level of speech not its fundamental object of investigation. Psychoanalysis is concerned with the unconscious signifying chain as its topological substratum and what jouissance is invoked or weaved for the reader by the localized brilliance of a necklace of metaphors and bright pearls.

The question of the relative importance of structure or signification versus jouissance in a text is also implicated in the aesthetic understanding of a text as a work of art. How much is a text a question of forces, magnitudes, and artistic beauty, versus a question of signifiers, and conceptual or logical structure. In addition, in literature, not only grammatical structure but also artistic style, or the way an author writes and/or tells a story, is important. Artistic style is what distinguishes one author from another and creates a unique voice for readers to hear.

In Lacanian analysis, style is also important for detecting the uniqueness of an author or a text. But style is more than simply an artistic feature. In the *Ecrits,* Lacan says that readers will know about his style by reading his text on "The Purloined Letter". "My style" here is a pun referring to both Lacan's style and Lacan's psychoanalytic definition of style. An easy entry into style is through understanding that the destination of the letter is always to be lost. This is how Y understand how "truth inhabits fiction". Truth inhabits fiction as causality in the form of a gap, or something missing within the structure of the signifier. The signifier designates propositional truth, but this truth can never fully manifest itself without the subject's own fictional misrecognition of his/her fate, and the narcissistic rationalization of this fate in his/her memory.

Lacan's writing style is unique, ornamented, and highly metaphorical. In the *Ecrits*, he uses this style to talk about style itself. Some readers take *Ecrits'* difficult writing style as Lacan's symptom or problem in writing. At best, Lacan's writing has been described or critiqued as being abstruse, obtuse, and cryptic, while, at worst, his writing has been parodied or ridiculed as incoherent, chaotic, and confused. Lacan's style is cryptic or obtuse because, like meaning, the letter and its destiny and destination is always to be lost, to be missing, and in absentia.

Literature is fiction because its truth is always missing or concealed and needs to be "read" and deciphered by the reader. Truth can never fully manifest itself without the subject's own fictional misrecognition of their fate, his/her identification with their "semblable", and secondarily without narcissistically conveniently rationalizing this fate in their memory. Self-reference, when the self in self-reference refers to the ego, is always highly problematical. When subjects lose themselves in the signifier, the reference is always metaphorical.

Yes, Lacan's style is his symptom, but, more than that, the symptom also shows Lacan's distinct approach to psychoanalysis and writing. In this sense, his style is also his sinthome. "The style is the man himself". The symptom represents the person, while the singularity is in the person. The sinthome is the person in himself/herself, and beyond himself. In literature, the example for a person of style is Oscar Wilde, who not only spoke and wrote about style, but also lived "his style" out.

In addition, the question of a person's style does not point to self-love and a person's narcissistic or histrionic "flair", as sometimes Lacan's style has been ridiculed. Like the formal signifier, style represents the subject, and leads away from the ego individual as the reference point. The perception of style is a question of style posed to the Other, and where the answer comes back to the subject in inverted form. The meaning of the statement "The man is the style" is heard backward. Paradoxically, or ironically, although man appears to be the focus, the actual reference is the style rather than the person.

Art, beauty, and style, all refer to questions of love and desire more than technical knowledge, although not exclusively. Literary theorists and psychoanalysts in general ask questions about both: what are the links among desire, stories, psychical structure, and formal knowledge about language?

> Since the point is to take desire, and since it can only be taken literally [a la lettre], since it is the letter's snare that determines, nay overdetermines, its place as a heavenly bird, how can we fail to require the bird catcher to first be a man of letters?
>
> (*Ecrits*, 2006, p. 536)

Desire cannot be found in ordinary speech acts. Desire is weaved at the letter level, the same level as the construction of the word itself. Lacan creatively uses the expression "man of letters" in the sense that the literary person, the writer, who gets us in contact with jouissance because jouissance structurally belongs to the letter. So, a jouissance of words or of the signifier could be only explained by the letter. For the Lacan of the Purloined Letter period, the real is the syntax underlying automaton, which is the ultimate reason of symbolic determination and yet cannot be fully symbolized in speech. For the later Lacan, it is the creative use of the letter within the Real unconscious (lalangue, or the language of the One) that generates jouissance.

The letter's snare overdetermines the apparent irrationality of desire, or its place as a bird of paradise, as Lacan says, and this is suggestive of satisfaction but also of suffering and loss. Loss of the beloved, or loss of love, is linked to how the letter comes to represent a hole in "the ardent place of the heart".

Writing and the letter is what infuses the Real of jouissance into psychical structure and the structure of a text. Since the letter is a basic unit of the signifier, breaking down words into letters in psychoanalysis is not that different from what Derrida said about deconstruction: "Deconstruction perhaps has the effect, if not the mission, of liberating forbidden jouissance" (Derrida, 1992, p. 65). Azari, p. 76. The sparks within the letters are released by the effect of deconstruction/interpretation.

What does it mean that the signifier leaves behind unsignified traces of the Real in the body, and that the Real of the body or the Mind writ large infuses the signifier and language with jouissance? How can you read the marks that clouds and raindrops leave on the ground other than as a mathematical measure of precipitation or the Real experience of being drenched by an influx of jouissance and precipitation? The writing of a cloud subject (*sujet sans substance*) brings to life the unthinkable and unsayable within a text.

Neither the Real nor the repressed unconscious lends themselves to symbolization without resistance. In the repressed unconscious resistance is a function of censorship and repression, while in the Real unconscious resistance is a function of the absolute difference between the Real and the Symbolic. The Real unconscious resists because its field lies outside the symbolic order. Such outside is both "ek-sistence" as an experience of jouissance and a topological or mathematical structure not easily convertible into language. Nevertheless, the Real unconscious of Lacan's later work transforms an incomplete universe of discourse into a field of jouissance.

The poetic function of language as conceived by Roman Jakobson is not different from how language works both within linguistic and unconscious mental structure as "lalangue" or the language of what the later Lacan calls the Real unconscious. In the Real unconscious links and associations are established through homophony, phonemes, and the sounds of the letters in language. Jakobson gives the example of a political slogan from the American presidential campaign of Dwight D. ("Ike") Eisenhower: "I like Ike". The I and Ike are repeated twice, and like and Ike are homophones. Through the homophonic link, the necessity of liking or the desire for Ike seems inscribed in the very structure of the language. As the phoneme was the basic unit of analysis for understanding the signifier and the repressed unconscious in the middle period of his work, homophony between phonemes becomes the basic unit of analysis for the Real unconscious of Lacan's later work.

The poetic function of language, as Lacan argues, and as demonstrated in this book, is also related to the way that metaphor is linked to the production of the subject and the cancellation of the imaginary ego. In a sense, psychoanalysis is both a science and a poetic art. The voice of a text is not the imaginary ego, but rather the I of the signifier that speaks for what otherwise would be an imaginary ego. The ego thinks that language advances the purposes and aims of the ego, while in actuality it is the pure signifier that advances and realizes the subject.

Finally, recent theorists, such as Kristeva, have argued for intertextuality or for the notion that works are made from other works that they take up, repeat, challenge, and transform. The notion of two or more texts and languages interacting is also found in psychical structure. The two forms of language interact with two modalities of mental structure: Psyche and Mind, desire, and defense. There are the laws of language, the language of the code and censorship, and then there is the language of desire and jouissance as its structural underside. Cs. Pcs. language interacts with the language of the unconscious, with sometimes one (Cs. Pcs.) representing the language of defense and the other, the language of desire and jouissance, while at other times the perspectives or the alignment between the two languages and the two aspect of psyche and mind are reversed. Sometimes the language of desire becomes a language of defense against jouissance so that desire can be reached through "the inverted ladder of the law".

This is a topological description of psychical reality. In speech there are always modalities and transformations acting upon letters, defenses, desires, and jouissance. So, the human Mind is always both logical and poetical, objective/abstract and subjective. That is why dyadic intersubjectivity cannot escape an imaginary fate, while the dialectical movements of signifiers are always beyond dualism, and sometimes beyond the Symbolic when the signified is located within a bodily experience of jouissance in the register of the Real.

In this sense, Moncayo (2012) has argued for a distinction between the Lacanian imaginary register and the human imagination. Imaginary does not mean literally untrue. The imaginary can also refer to the imagination or to what is visionary or inventive. Lacan says that truth is half-fiction, half-imaginary, or we could say half-ideological. However, up to this point Lacanian theory has still left untheorized the further question of an Imagination or an imaginative faculty that reveals new images within the field of vision that, despite being subjective, give an accurate depiction of reality. The Imaginary may be consistent with ideology (although not entirely), but the imagination is not. The Lacanian imaginary also provides a theory with which to understand ideology so it cannot be simply reduced to being a form of false knowledge or cogito.

As Moncayo has pointed out, many scientific discoveries have been described through the categories of the positive imagination as a kind of light dawning experience. Moncayo mentioned the examples of Mendeleyev who dreamt the periodic table of elements; of Einstein who rode a beam of light to its logical conclusion; Newton who daydreamed about a falling apple, and Darwin who, when the theory of evolution hit him, he said it seemed as if the scales fell from his eyes. Finally, Gutenberg described the idea of the printing press as coming like a beam of light, and another physicist was daydreaming in a London bus when suddenly he saw atoms falling into molecules. All these images reveal more than hide the relations between the elements of a structure. Here images and the elements of the Imagination provide a perspective by which a new logic can be fathomed.

Another way to understand the difference between the Imaginary and the Imagination is to use the logic of the three registers where a two-way relationship between the Imaginary and the Symbolic can be established. The Imaginary represents an Imaginary use of the Symbolic or I/S, and the Imagination represents a Symbolic use of the Imaginary or S/I. The Imaginary use of the Symbolic constitutes the apparent opposition between appearance and reality or the way that the Imaginary of objective reality appears to function independently and in disregard of symbolic determination and subjectivity. With respect to fantasy life or fiction, the Imaginary attempts to fill in or conceals the gaps or the lack within the Symbolic. Fantasies as imaginary configurations of the Symbolic are to be differentiated from Symbolic uses of the Imaginary and the Real. Flashes of insight or great moments of discovery constitute Symbolic uses of the Imaginary to represent the Real.

The categories of the creative imagination are a function of the hole within the Symbolic to represent the Real. Creative images emerge out of the navel of the Symbolic that opens out into the unknown or the unseen structure of being. We have to see with the eye of the Symbolic in order to correct the normal imaginary distortion of vision and use the creative imagination to arrive at new visions of reality via permutations of the symbolic structure.

References

Azari, E. (2008). Lacan and the Destiny of Literature. London: Continuum.
Lacan, J. (2006). Ecrits. New York: Norton & Norton.
Derrida, J. (1992). On an apocalyptic tone newly adopted in philosophy. In: Derrida and Negative Theology. New York: State University of New York Press.
Moncayo, R, (2012). The emptiness of Oedipus. London: Routledge.
Rabate, J.M. (2014). The Cambridge Introduction to Literature and Psychoanalysis. Cambridge: Cambridge University Press.

Chapter 3

History of Modern English, Literary Theory, and Lacanian Psychoanalysis

Literature theory nowadays is one of the fields where the creative traditional values of English society, compromised by industrial capitalism, can be investigated and explored. In the past 200 years, the British Empire provided a big impetus to the development of industrial capitalism in England as well as vice versa.

From this point of view, literature and modern English use are explicitly ideological. Writing embodies the values and tastes of a particular social class. According to Eagleton (2003) the development of English studies is directly proportional to the decline or failure of religion in the modern world. The Victorian ruling class was very concerned and alarmed by the decline of religion as a civilizing force. Literature was seen as an alternative modern discourse to replace and provide a displaced version of the virtues associated with religion (humility, altruism, and reflection).

But English was not only construed as an alternative to religion. Despite the fact that English has become the language of science, English was also constructed as an alternative to the modern science that society was erecting as the model of true knowledge but that left much to be desired as far as the psychical and emotional constitution of the civil subject is concerned. Like religion before, English literature, as a socializing influence different from natural science and the science of evolution, needed to organize sexual and aggressive impulses without too much repression, conflict, or frustration.

We argue that psychoanalysis as a discourse is in between the use of language or ideology as an alternative to religion and the natural sciences, which, beyond objective knowledge, don't have much to offer society as an alternative to religion. Psychoanalysis is a social science that is neither solely literature nor an exact natural science but that addresses many of the social and mental ills previously addressed by religion.

While psychoanalysis addresses social and individual disorders, it does not establish ideological norms either for treatment or for theory. In this psychoanalysis differs from literary theory, political theory, and also religion. However, psychoanalysis has, will, and should influence theory in the humanities and social sciences. On the other hand, psychoanalytic theory should also update itself by using theory from adjacent fields. This is precisely what Freud and Lacan did and characterizes their work.

DOI: 10.4324/9781003424574-3

Finally, after Freud and Lacan, neither should anyone construe religion as a treatment for mental disorders, nor should religion's purpose be reduced to or used for the secular treatment of social disorders. Literature, politics, and religion are ideological forms, and therefore can be competing ideologies, although not necessarily. It is not for psychoanalytic theory to determine their relative merits since this would be an ideological function. Instead, psychoanalysis can serve to illuminate the mental and symbolic structures embedded within these fields. In this book we intend to do precisely that. We intend to find the mental and symbolic structures embedded in the text, not only to develop psychoanalytic theory, but also because this approach may throw some modest light on the interpretation of the text (although this is not our main intent), and at the same time may help develop the field of literary studies.

In the twentieth-century era of modern psychological man, literature, according to some, has become a whole alternative ideology and a whole new way (however successful or unsuccessful it may be) of socializing the civic individual. However, the psychological man within the context of the liberal individual and society can also represent the isolated and atomized individual of capitalism. The notion of a self-interested and isolated liberal and capitalist individual is only an egoic or imaginary notion of a subject.

On the one hand, the subject, as a signifier, is a collectivity, while the subject in the Real of jouissance is something else. What Lacan calls the ego in the Real is Lacan's (1971–1972) subject "All-alone", or Winnicott's (1963) "true isolate", that, according to Lacan, appears in the place of the lack of sexual rapport between the sexes. There is no rapport between the sexes because of the fantasy that always involves the two. When the subject abandons the pursuit of the fantasy other, then the subject is All-Alone, but not necessarily lonely. Lacan's term "All-alone" may be related to the "I" in ancient China? The emperor called himself 孤meaning alone, 寡人, Person alone/the singular person. But Lacan adds "All" in front of "alone" for emphasis.

The subject All-alone does not represent a failure in object or social relatedness but rather a healthy, benevolent, and satisfying form of solitude and aloneness that includes relationships, and in fact facilitates the possibility that relationships may in fact work out after all. Lacan's subject All-alone, however, is "not-All One whole Being", for also it is naught/not. That the Real subject is "All-alone" also means that in the Symbolic the subject is "not-All alone". The subject (as signifier) is a collectivity within the Symbolic. But within the Real the subject is All-alone, despite being many at the level of the signifier. From many One, and from One many, as stated in the motto of the United States (derived from Heraclitus' tenth fragment).

According to modern literary theory, literature as a phenomenon has existed for more than 2,000 years (beginning with Biblical stories), while literature as a concept began to develop since the Romantic period. The whole point of creative writing and a liberal education was that it was useless or at least not oriented toward economic profit. Mass technological culture is not the inevitable product of industrial society, but of a particular form of profit- or gain-oriented industrialism and consumerism that centered production around profit rather than use, or around fantasy rather than the Real (empty) value of things. Literature, from this perspective, becomes a romantic protest against the mechanized slavery, oppressiveness, and cultural poverty of capitalism.

In this way, according to Eagleton (1983), English literature acquires a triple function. Eagleton mentions three functions but then names four, an accident that is consistent with the function of the topological knot of four used by Lacan. In our words, and from this perspective, literature educates, delights, provides a cure for the psyche, and heals the state. Healing the state, of course, would be an ideological function.

For many critics and writers of the late nineteenth and early twentieth century, the urgent social need was to educate or cultivate the materialistic middle class. The influence of Greek culture here is not accidental and coincided with Joyce's desire to Hellenize the English language (*L'Elanges*). With Greek culture represented by Helen, Lacan literalizes the question by punning on the homophony of "El". "El" represents the educating or enlightening aspect of language or of the word. However, when this educating aspect becomes formalized, the playful or jouissance value of speech becomes truncated or underdeveloped. Joyce wants to Hellenize English but in a Dionysian rather than Apollonian style. For the same yet different reason, Lacan wants to go in the opposite direction from the Latin, to the Greek root of the word sinthome. In the old version, the symptom, or suffering, was also linked to saintliness. This aspect of the symptom is lost in the modern use of the word symptom.

State-established schools, as Eagleton notes, by linking the middle and working classes to the best culture of their nation, will confer on them a great noble spirit. The middle class or the educated working class had to take over from the aristocracy the noble task of educating the working classes. Through education all people and things acquire a natural form of grace and nobility.

In this sense literature deals with universal human values but does this fact inevitably make English or language an ideology as Eagleton believes. If English helps to promote agreement and fellow feeling among all classes, from an ancient spiritual or cultural perspective, literature opens a serene and luminous dimension of truth as jouissance or the "heart" of the signifier. This is what Benjamin (1921) also called an unalloyed agreement between people.

Such light of satisfaction is not to distract from the satisfaction of material needs, but rather place them in their proper non-materialistic perspective. Biological and social needs are met but this is not confused with the satisfaction of desire which is something impossible that needs to be handled according to a different discourse associated both with language and with psychical structure. The satisfaction of desire requires the lack and emptiness as a constructive element of culture and of symbolic production and reproduction. This should not be confused with an ideology that covertly tells people to expect a deficit in the satisfaction of their basic biological and social needs.

When desire is addressed through literature and writing, students of literature occupy the more psychical territory of feeling and experience associated with desire. Does this mean that English as culture is associated more with science and objective knowledge rather than ideology? Is subjectivity or language always ideological? Precisely, psychoanalysis constitutes a science of subjectivity that is subjective, and yet a science insofar as it differentiates between imaginary and fantasized subjective idiosyncrasies, and a more objective use of language as a mathematical structure. From the point of view of the signifier, and its associated delights, literature and language become what Eagleton calls a sublime civilizing pursuit, or what we would call the "empty spiritual essence" of the social formation. Although as we shall demonstrate in Chapter 2, Henry James' work was not without controversy in this respect, people could at least have the fantasy that by reading Henry James they could become a better person, if not one of the "elites".

The conservative alternative to what is being presented is represented by T. S. Eliot, for whom the European Tradition of Mind represented a conservative alternative to a middle-class liberal education for the masses. However, liberal education is an ideology whereas Lacanian psychoanalysis we argue is not. A chauvinistic European tradition as a form of colonialism is also an ideology. The European tradition of Mind has evolved to the present in the form of Lacanian psychoanalysis which does not constitute an ideology because the totalizing imaginary defenses and deceptions linked to ideology have been interpreted and deconstructed thanks to a new discourse, and to a new understanding regarding the nature of perception.

What was needed to construct a non-ideological and secular function for language was the evolution of a sensory language and discourse which could establish an internal dialogue with the mind, the body, and the brain. Paraphrasing Eliot (1920), "the tentacular roots of words" need to reach not only to other metonymical signifiers of desire in the net of language and mind, but also to signifieds residing within the body, as well as semiotic signs at work within the nervous system and the brain. The signifier suggests enigmatic images that penetrate to the most primitive and original levels of human experience.

Literature should be a solution to social problems, not part of them or of the ideology that keeps them in place. The poem and the flower must be plucked free from the oppressive chains of history and elevated to the dignity of das Ding (the "thing" or "no-thing"), as Lacan says.

A psychoanalytic, critical, and scientific account of literature investigates the ambiguities, tensions, paradoxes, and ambivalences at play in the structure of language. As is well known, European history in the twentieth century celebrated the decentering of the subject linked to Darwin, Freud, and Marx. The human being is no longer in control of his/her destiny, and instead is ruled by unconscious evolutionary, instinctual, and social forces. Phenomenology, and North American ego psychology in reaction, restored the transcendental or autonomous ego to the center position it previously occupied ever since the Italian renaissance.

But since psychoanalysis is a modern discourse, the deferment of signification to the signifier cannot represent a simple regression to the prepossession held by traditional authority. After all, the ego for Freud was connatural to the idea of rational critique, progress, and emancipation. With Lacanian theory we are faced with the challenge of linking a modern critical tradition associated with the agency of reason, to the Lacanian notion of the subject as a metaphor.

The deferment of signification to the signifier represents a deferment of signification to the subject rather than the ego. But does the subject have its own voice or only speaks with the words of the Other? Does the subject simply represent a subjection to the Other's desire, as was the case in the Middle Ages around the globe? The answer to this riddle comes from the side of desire. We cannot speak of a deferment of signification to the signifier without, at the same time, raising the question of the subject's singular desire as different from the Other's desire.

When the signifier represents the subject, the subject is represented by a signifier of desire. It is the signifier of desire that leads to the question of individual choice, authenticity, and responsibility when it comes to speech and human action. At the same time, human desire, and a subject's desire, is represented by the signifier that comes from the Other. The relative autonomy of desire is one of interdependence rather than opposition to the signifier.

In addition, desire is singular, and every analysis is one by one. The dimension of the One cannot be eliminated, even when it is the signifier that represents the subject and at the same time misrepresents the subject of jouissance or desire. The dimension of the One is not represented by the ego that appropriates or clings to the signifier. The unity of the One is Real, while the ego's unity is Imaginary. Ego autonomy is not the same as the One jouissance of the subject of the Real that takes responsibility for his/her desire.

When it is the ego that advances the self and the signifier, rather than metaphor or the signifier that advances the subject, then this is also the figure of the false egotistical leader of a group or the faceless masses. The human spirit instead arises in the gap between nonmeaning and meaning, and in between the ego and the subject. The pure signifier cannot in truth be embodied in a human subject without the subject mourning the inexistant imaginary phallus and surrendering the power of ego domination to the power of metaphor and the signifier.

Literature for Heidegger (1953, pp. 347–389) was a "Way" to experience what happens in history and in the symbolic structure that turns it into authentically meaningful experience that advances and illuminates the subject. Is experience simply intellectually meaningful, or does human experience also provide a way to reconcile the conflicts between desire and culture, or between desire and the desire of the Other? According to psychoanalysis, simply by reading literature, subjects cannot take responsibility for their desires.

Thus, contemporary literature marks a transition from the preoccupation with the author in Romanticism, to an exclusive concern with the text in modern criticism, as seen in Lacan's text, to a marked shift of attention to the reader, which, in our opinion, refers to the function of psychoanalysis, and psychical structure, not literature theory per se. Lacan's textual analysis always refers back to the practice of analysis and the focus on the reader does not signal a return to the transcendental ego as the locus of explanation. Lacan did not think psychoanalysts should interpret an author's work by reducing it to their biographical historical narratives or conscious "psychological dynamics".

A letter or text belongs to an author, but once written, the text/letter belongs to the holder or reader of a text, or the reader as the holder and enunciator of a text in the continuous present moment. We agree with Lacan and modern criticism that a text or the symbolic order is independent from the subject, and therefore the focus on the reader could also be misplaced. It is the reading and the subjective position of the reader that really matters and functions.

The shift to the author can be observed in Barthes' (1975) text, "The Pleasure of the Text". For Barthes the death of the author is a place of jouissance or of the death drive within the text.

> The text you write must prove to me that it desires me. This proof exists: it is writing. Writing is: the science of the various blisses of language, its Kama Sutra (this science has but one treatise, writing itself). Language reconstructs itself elsewhere under the teeming flux of every kind of linguistic pleasure.
>
> (p. 8)

Although Literature can be said to represent a cognitive construct because it yields a knowledge of the world, by the same token it has also been defined as a form of utopian dreaming about fundamental human desires and their objects. Beyond bondage and determinism, literature is the one place where fantasy can appear to fly free despite the fact that such flight has to be looped within a language structure and, of course, in language, censorship is inescapable. In fiction desires appear to be acted out through the characters of a story.

However, this kind of freedom does not represent free association for psychoanalysis. Free association involves conjuring up the repressed but not necessarily acting it out, since free association and "J'ouis-sense" (analytical listening to the significance of speech) lead to symbolization and not necessarily to acting out. Free association requires equal attention to desire and lack, and to the desire that is reached through the inverted ladder of the law. After going up or down the inverted ladder of the law, subjects may decide if what they want is really what they want and take responsibility for it. Otherwise, the so-called freedom of desire is in fact Utopian illusory dreaming about a human desire that cannot be fulfilled. Working with human desire requires a narrow psychoanalytic path beyond the illusion of complete fulfillment, and the ascesis represented by the repression of human desire. The satisfaction of desire differs from the realistic satisfaction of necessary and legitimate human needs.

A reader is expected not only to experience pleasure and relief in relationship to a text but to use various cultural and symbolic codes to elucidate it (Eco, 1979). Literary theory's shift of attention to the reader means that signifiers "have to reflect inward experiences or objects in the real world, and to make present the subject's own thoughts and feelings about reality" (Eagleton, p. 112).

However, a psychoanalytic reading differs from an ideological reading of a text. The meaning of the linguistic and mathematical structure that organizes the symbolic order cannot be reduced to binary dualistic categories erected by ego-based social masters to benefit the interests of patriarchy or the oligarchy. The narrative or telling of the story is the Imaginary but the structure is a symbolic system or a battery of signifiers that exceeds the doings of social subjects without this representing or being misconstrued as a malevolent form of alienation. A text is a window to the universal human mind embodied in symbolic structure.

A psychoanalytic reading of a text is not ideological. A psychoanalytic reading does not seek to actively promote social family values, explicit forms of authority, or the liberal values of independence, liberty, and democracy. Derrida (1976) fails to understand Lacan and the meaning of the phallus as the signifier of a lack. Instead, Derrida and feminism read the meaning of the phallus in the Imaginary as a signifier of privilege or masculine supremacy. When women are seen as being assigned a negative value in relation to the male-first principle, this analysis misunderstands the nature of the imaginary phallus.

The presence and absence of the imaginary phallus is misread by Derrida as Lacan's "phallocentrism" and "logocentrism" or "logophallocentrism". Our position is that Derrida and Lacan are not that far apart, and when they are it is because Derrida misunderstands Lacan, and misunderstands or ignores the function of the Real and Lacan's later work. The presence of the phi for imaginary masculinity represents a necessary provisional illusion at best, and the same goes for its absence in the case of imaginary femininity. Both presence and absence in the Imaginary are re-signified in the Symbolic. Men have to lose and grieve the imaginary phallus, while women have to realize its inexistence, and it is this realization that inscribes the feminine into the symbolic structure. The center or fixed principle here is not the imaginary presence of an erect phallus but a true hole of Real jouissance that orients the symbolic structure.

In "The Purloined Letter", Lacan asks whether the Symbolic is organized by causal determination or by arbitrary chance factors. Lacan clearly considers chance as an organizing factor for the symbolic order. Derrida misses this when, in his critique of Lacan, he thinks that Lacan does not consider chance and only thinks of symbolic structure as fixated on a transcendental signifier of the phallus as a privileged presence.

Chance factors refer to the concept of the repetition compulsion at work within the structure of the signifier, although automaton represents a moment of maximum determination that only appears to be purely accidental. "My research has led me to the realization that repetition automatism (*Wiederholungs wang*) has its basis in what I have called the insistence of the signifying chain". Is the insistence of the signifying chain always about a surplus form of phallic jouissance or phallic signifier/object? Thus, in the opening chapter we ask the question whether the repetition compulsion is ruled by a principle of causal determination or by an aleatory chance principle since Lacan seems to be alluding to both. Is the chance combination of signifiers the mainspring of equivocation in the unconscious?

Freud (1920) gave the example of traumatic accidental factors that overwhelmed the defensive barriers of the ego. The excessive intensities and symptoms generated by the trauma continue to repeat in an effort to master, reduce, and calm the painful excitations. Freud gave many examples of how people repeat the same patterns in relationships, births, deaths, accidents, and traumas as their parents. In addition, there are the unintended repetitions of group conflicts, social problems with leaders, and historical events ever since time immemorial. Finally, we will argue that causal determination, and the repetition compulsion, can appear as a chance factor, while Tyche is the true principle of "*un*determination", healing, and change.

Poe's story provoked a debate among literary theorists in the 1960s and 1970s with other authors, and Parisian intellectual peers of Lacan, offering other interpretations of Poe's text than those set forth by Lacan. It is not the purpose of this chapter to offer yet another additional interpretation of the text, nor shall we follow the same literary analytic method used by Lacan. The purpose of the chapter is not simply to review and critique what other Lacanian authors have said about the story and provide yet another interpretation, however accurate it may be.

We will consider the theory that Lacan proposed in the text, and contrast it with his later theoretical developments, in particular his theory of the Real and of jouissance. Does the analysis of the text change with the later theory of various jouissances that Lacan proposes?

This book is not about the writer but more about the use that Lacanian theory makes of a writer's story, not to apply psychoanalysis to a literary subject, although Lacan certainly does that in his paper, but rather to use the literary text to guide the itinerary and direction of psychoanalytic and Lacanian theory as a mode of discourse and signifying practice.

In this chapter we will use Lacan's text, and Lacan's reading of Poe's text, to test Lacan's later theory of the Real and jouissance, much like Lacan did with Joyce. We will argue that the Suite, which was also written at the time of the Purloined Letter text, possesses a logic of its own, stemming from logic and mathematics that provides an underlying structure for the theory of the signifier and fantasy life. Consistent with these principles, the analysis of The Turn of the Screw in Chapter 4 will be focused on a detailed analysis of Lacan's Seminar XIV on the Logic of the Fantasy.

For his part Norman Holland (1968) sees literature as a function of the subjective interplay of unconscious fantasies and conscious defenses against them. Reading a literary work is enjoyable because reading a text in this view is an emotionally transformative experience. A historically relevant text helps the subject transform the anxieties and fears associated with desire. This is solely a conventional adaptive function of reading and literature. Here literature functions as a kind of release valve or psychotherapeutic relief that makes the repressive structure more bearable. However, the origin and the reason for repression are structural, while also having historical effects. In other words, anxieties linked to unconscious fantasies cannot be prevented by moral hygiene or a lessening of social repressions.

Literature and reading can be a form of therapy like exercise, socialization, and entertainment but this is not psychoanalysis. In addition, many binary oppositions, such as light and dark, or material form and vacuum, cannot be deconstructed, as Derrida suggests, because they and Nature are not the fabrications of a human ego agency associated with a patriarchal or a historically determined capitalist form of social organization.

The transformative practices of psychoanalysis are not the same as the radical politics associated with a confusion among need, demand, and desire that mistakes the realization of human desire with a desire for political emancipation, or the overcoming of social oppression as being the same as the undoing of psychical repression in the psychoanalytic process.

This form of understanding collapses the distinction between the psychical and the sociological. Psychical repression is necessary for healthy subjectivity and civilization and is absolutely not the same as historically determined forms of social oppression. Not that politics needs to be ignored, but that symbolic structure should not be confused with oppression or a political manifesto. Symbolic acts, just like language or mental structure, are not necessarily political or ideological. Ideology represents the imaginary impregnations or "cover" of the symbolic structure. Contrary to what Eagleton argues, literary theory is not political in this sense, and Lacanian psychoanalysis cannot be reduced to being a convenient device for the ideological apparatus of the modern capitalist state. The main function of psychoanalysis is not to support conventional identities; instead, Lacan's paternal/parental metaphor supports the necessary psychical and family structure that cannot be reduced or confounded with the structure of malevolent forms of patriarchal organization.

By a better understanding of the pleasures and displeasures readers experience in literature and life in general, a modest but significant light may be cast on the question of human suffering.

Finally, Lacanian psychoanalysis and its "cure" of human suffering do not represent a repressive "transcendence" of the drive, desire, or the material world, nor its fulfillment, but through insight and realization, the drive, pure desire, and the vacuum may in fact become liberating for the subject. Repressive transcendence or de-sublimation mean opposite things. Repressive transcendence, for example, means transforming anger through controlling and repressing it.

References

Benjamin, W. (1996). *Critique of Violence*. Cambridge: The Belknap Press of Harvard University Press. P. 236–252

Eagleton, T. (2003). *Literary Theory*. Minneapolis: The University of Minnesota.

Eco, H. (1979). *The Role of the Reader. Explorations in the Semiotics of Texts*. Bloomington: Indiana University Press, 1984.

Eliot, T. S. (1920). *The Sacred Wood*. New York: Alfred A. Knopf, 1921.

Derrida, J. (1976). *Of Grammatology*. Baltimore, MD: John Hopkins University Press.

Eagleton, T. (1983). *Literary Theory*. Oxford: Blackwell.

Freud, S. (1920). Beyond the Pleasure Principle. *SE*, 18, 7–64.

Heidegger, M. (1953). *Being and Time*. New York: State University of New York Press.

Holland, N. (1968). *The Dynamics of Literary Response*. New York: Oxford University Press.

Lacan, J. (1971–1972). *...ou pire (Or Worse)*. Book XIX. Unpublished translation by C. Gallagher. www.lacaninireland.com.

Rimmon-Kenan, S. (1987). *Discourse in Psychoanalysis and Literature*. London: Routledge.

Winnicott, R. (1963). *New Library of Psychoanalysis Teaching Series*. Edited by Birksted-Breen, Dana; Lesley Caldwell; Angela Joyce. London: Karnac Books.

Chapter 4

The Itinerary and Destiny of the Letter

With the Purloined Letter text Lacan intended to illustrate certain truths that he drew out of the body of Freud's work. From Freud, Lacan derives the thesis that it is the symbolic order which is constitutive for the subject. The signifier is preeminent over the subject and over the signified. By his analysis of Poe's text Lacan wants to demonstrate how the subject is determined by what he calls the itinerary of the signifier. It is the truths of desire embedded in the signifying structure that through a series of substitutions and secondary elaborations are represented in a story, or a fictional piece of literature.

In his text, Lacan performs a step-by-step literary analysis of the narrative by first presenting some key concepts of psychoanalysis, followed by an analysis of the logic of the text, which is interpreted according to psychoanalytic principles.

Lacan believed that an analytic and literary analysis of the coherence of any story or fable can bring to light the signifying structure of desire embedded within a work of literary fiction. Lacan wants to bring out the unnoticed coherence or the underlying logic running through a text or story. Lacan moves from scenes to subjects and characters, and from characters to letters as both objects and signifiers.

In addition, in this text Lacan raises the question whether the Symbolic is organized by causal determination or by arbitrary chance factors. Chance factors refer to the concept of the repetition compulsion at work within the structure of the signifier. "My research has led me to the realization that repetition automatism (Wiederholungs wang) has its basis in what I have called the insistence of the signifying chain" (Ecrits, 2006). Thus, in this opening chapter we ask the question whether the repetition compulsion is ruled by a principle of causal determination or by an aleatory chance principle since Lacan seems to be alluding to both. Is the chance combination of signifiers the mainspring of equivocation in the unconscious? Finally, we will argue that causal determination, and the repetition compulsion, can appear as a chance factor, while Tyche is the true principle of *un*determination, healing, and change.

Poe's story provoked a debate among literary theorists in the 1960s and 1970s with other authors, and Parisian intellectual peers of Lacan, offering other interpretations of Poe's text than those set forth by Lacan. It is not the purpose of this chapter to offer yet another additional interpretation of the text, nor shall we follow the

DOI: 10.4324/9781003424574-4

same literary analytic method used by Lacan. Lacan begins his text by introducing relevant analytic concepts that will be employed for the study of the text, and then continues with a page-by-page analysis of the text interspersed with an elucidation of psychoanalytic ideas that could help carry the analysis of the text further. My method is different, and the purpose of the chapter is not simply to review and critique what other Lacanian authors have said about the story and provide yet another interpretation, however accurate it may be.

We will consider the theory that Lacan proposed in the text, and contrast it with his later theoretical developments, in particular his theory of the Real and of jouissance. Would the analysis of the text change with the later theory of jouissance? In the Ecrits Lacan introduces the concept of jouissance as something inconvenient, deadly, and traumatic that breaks the shield and barrier set up by the pleasure principle to protect the subject from unpleasant or painful experiences. When the protective barrier is breached, when tensions reach a certain magnitude or threshold, the subject experiences pain rather than pleasure.

However, jouissance not only represents the point where pleasure turns into unpleasure. Jouissance is also used by Lacan to represent a form of phallic enjoyment as a form of pleasure or satisfaction (Lacan speaks of masturbatory jouissance whether penile or clitoral – both of which are figures for the imaginary phallus). Here we already observe two different forms of jouissance, both of which can be pleasant and/or unpleasant. Phallic jouissance can be unpleasant due to the imaginary identifications associated to "having" or "not-having" the imaginary phallus. That is to say, narcissistic imaginations and identifications can hardly be avoided in phallic jouissance.

The jouissance of the Other represents the fusion with the mother and the fantasy of the imaginary phallus. The fusion with the mother is initially necessary but at some point it becomes inconvenient without the intervention of the Other that turns the jouissance of the Other into phallic jouissance. Phallic jouissance is pleasant and convenient, so long as it is ruled by symbolic castration. On the other hand, the imaginary phallus, as an attribute of the father, also plays a necessary function in facilitating the transition from the first to the second jouissance, and from the first to the second phase of Oedipus.

However, if the phallus remains in an imaginary fantasized position and becomes reified, this leads to an endless search for surplus phallic jouissance that eventually also becomes inconvenient or destructive. It is the fantasy of the inexistent imaginary phallus that drives the search for surplus jouissance. The imaginary phallus has to be revealed as inexistant, for the symbolic phallus to function as an organizing principle of the Symbolic that also gives access to the Real as the outside – the signifier (lack of a signifier for the Real). The symbolic phallus is the signifier of a lack rather than a positive privilege.

In the *Ecrits* Lacan had not elaborated the relationship between a symptom as a metaphor and as a form of jouissance. "For the symptom is a metaphor, whether one likes to admit it or not, just as desire is a metonymy, even if man scoffs at the idea". The symptom here is a ciphered message.

> From 1962 on, there is a gradual tendency in Lacan's work away from the linguistic conception of the symptom, and towards a view of the symptom as pure jouissance which cannot be interpreted. This conceptual shift culminates in 1975 with the introduction of the term sinthome.

For the later Lacan symptoms can no longer be entirely resolved by interpretation or an analysis of symbols and language. Symptoms depend on factors that lie outside language and the Symbolic. With the concept of the sinthome, Lacan redefines the psychoanalytic symptom in terms of his final topology of the subject.

> "In 1963 Lacan goes on to state that the symptom does not call for interpretation; since in itself, it is not a call to the Other but a pure jouissance addressed to no one (Lacan, 1962–3: seminar of 23 January 1963; see Miller, 1987:11)." The symptom is how the subject enjoys the unconscious.
>
> This move from conceiving of the symptom as a message which can be deciphered by reference to the unconscious "structured like a language", to seeing it as the trace of the particular modality of the subject's jouissance, culminates in the introduction of the term sinthome. The sinthome thus designates a signifying formulation beyond analysis, a kernel of enjoyment immune to the efficacy of the symbolic. Far from calling for some analytic "dissolution", the sinthome is what "allows one to live" by providing a unique organization of jouissance. The task of analysis thus becomes, in one of Lacan's last definitions of the end of analysis, to identify with the sinthome.
>
> (p.189)

The concept of the sinthome makes it possible to study jouissance beyond language or discourse analysis which is inevitably interweaved with the Symbolic. This is also why the later Lacan puts emphasis on the Real and goes more and more into the abstract mathematical world. The sinthome is beyond meaning and therefore it is not completely analyzable. In Joyce's epiphanies the Real forecloses meaning. The symbolic order is invaded by jouissance. Jouissance represents a new way of using language. Free association leads to an experience of jouissance in relationship to signifiers more than to abstract intellectual analysis embedded in a narcissistic ego structure.

This chapter is not about Poe the writer, but more about the use that Lacan makes of Poe's story, not to apply psychoanalysis to a literary subject, although he certainly does that in his paper, but rather to use the literary text to illustrate the itinerary and direction of psychoanalytic and Lacanian theory. Lacan did not think psychoanalysts should interpret an author's work by reducing it to their biographical historical narratives or "psychological dynamics". In our case, and for purposes of this chapter, we will use Lacan's text, and Lacan's reading of Poe's text, to test Lacan's later theory of the Real and jouissance, much like Lacan did with Joyce.

Lacan uses Poe's text to illustrate the theory of the Symbolic order that he had at the time. This is particularly the case with the Suite at the end of the text that has been rarely read and commented upon. We will argue that the Suite, which was also written at the time of the Purloined Letter text, possesses a logic of its own, stemming from logic and mathematics that provides an underlying structure for the theory of the signifier.

Finally, a psychoanalytic reading of a literary text in no way presumes that a writer's work can be limited to psychoanalytic or Lacanian ideas. A psychoanalytic reading of a literary text may help a literary scholar develop theory within their own respective fields of study, or it could lead them to the study of the theory and practice of psychoanalysis as a supplementary field of research and investigation.

To this effect this chapter will consist of five sections described below. The first two focus on the analysis of the literary text itself, its structure and inner coherence, followed by a psychoanalytic and Lacanian reading of the story. The third section will stress the development of Lacanian theory over time (from the middle to the final period, and from the Symbolic to the Real). The last two sections will put to use the new theory of the Real and jouissance in the analysis and understanding of both Lacan's and Poe's text as a function of an interaction between the signifier and the letter, between the letter and the Real of jouissance.

1 The first section will consist of a brief summary of the plot of Poe's story. This section is included for the reader's convenience, and although it outlines the structure of the plot, perhaps in novel ways, the plot summary itself is not new and is widely available for anyone to read.
2 The summary of the plot will be followed by a survey of how Poe's text was understood by different philosophers and literary scholars in the past decades.
3 The third section will place sections of the Purloined Letter text in the larger context of the scope and history of Lacanian theory in order to demonstrate the transition from the middle period to the final period of Lacan's theory centered around the Real and the Borromean knot of four.
4 The fourth section considers the Suite at the end of the Purloined Letter text to show how Lacan attempts to develop a theory of the Symbolic in its relationship to logic and mathematics and how The Purloined Letter text and The Suite are related to each other.
5 The final section will discuss the relationship between the letter and the signifier, and the transition from logic and principia mathematica (PM system) to topology, from the signifier to jouissance, and from automaton to Tyche as two different forms of chance, one false and one true. Automaton is false as a form of chance, while representing a true form of psychical causality and overdetermination. Tyche instead is truly undetermined and acausal as a form of chance.

Plot Summary

The unnamed narrator is with the famous Parisian amateur detective C. Auguste Dupin when they are joined by G., prefect of the Paris police. The Prefect has a case he would like to discuss with Dupin.

A letter from the queen's lover has been stolen from her boudoir by the unscrupulous Minister D. D was in the room, saw the letter, and switched it for a letter of no importance. He has been blackmailing the queen.

The prefect makes two deductions with which Dupin does not disagree:

1 The contents of the letter have not been revealed, as this would have led to certain circumstances that have not arisen. The circumstances that have not arisen refers to the suffering and social scandal (inconvenient jouissance) that the letter would represent for the royal family, the government, and the nation. Forbidden phallic jouissance becomes a source of suffering for the Queen, and potentially for the King as well, because Minister D still has the letter in his possession. Forbidden phallic jouissance also implies that the forbidden aspect of the fantasy makes phallic jouissance function as the jouissance of the Other that is always greener on the other side, if only it was not forbidden, or precisely because it is forbidden.

   The symbolic order, as embodied in the King, the Queen, Dupin, and the structure of the signifier, is attempting to prevent that the Queen's indiscretions (phallic enjoyment) devolve into destructive forms of the perverse jouissance of the Other. The symbolic order needs to maintain a certain consistency for the structure.

2 The ability to produce the letter at a moment's notice is almost as important as actual possession of the letter. Therefore, he must have the letter close at hand.

The prefect says that he and his police detectives have searched the Minister's town house and have found nothing. Dupin asks the prefect if he knows what he is seeking, and the prefect reads a minute description of the letter (the searching of the letter involves the possibility that the letter would become known to everybody if the police found the letter), which Dupin memorizes (Dupin knows the content, but the Queen is his friend, and the prefect works for the Queen). The prefect then bids them good day.

Regarding this section of the story Lacan comments that:

> The first dialogue – between the Prefect of Police and Dupin – is played as if it were between a deaf man and one who hears. That is, it presents the veritable complexity of what is ordinarily simplified, with the most confused of results, in the notion of communication.

For Lacan due to the logical structure embedded in language (the true is preceded by the false, as revealed in the logic of material implication examined in the next chapter), and the metonymic structure of the Symbolic, every communication in language is a form of miscommunication and misunderstanding.

The text continues and a month later the prefect returns, still unsuccessful in his search. He is motivated to continue his fruitless search by the promise of a large reward, recently doubled, upon the letter's safe return, and he will pay 50,000 francs to anyone who can help him. Dupin asks him to write that check now and he will give him the letter. The prefect is astonished but knows that Dupin is not joking. Dupin induces the prefect to write the check with a miser's example, and Dupin produces the letter. The prefect determines that it is genuine and races to deliver it to the queen.

Alone together, the narrator asks Dupin how he found the letter. Dupin explains the Paris police are competent within their limitations but have underestimated with whom they are dealing. The prefect mistakes the Minister D for a fool because he is a poet. The prefect takes D for a common criminal, while Dupin (who is duped only up to a point) understands that what is at stake is the poetic and metaphoric structure of language and letters themselves. Metaphor, as explored in a subsequent chapter, manages to cross over and overcome the bar of social and unconscious censorship in language, and produce a metaphor that conceals yet also reveals the structure of the story and of poetic language.

Here Dupin explains how an eight-year-old boy made a small fortune from his friends at a game called Odds and Evens. The boy had determined the intelligence of his opponents and played upon that to interpret their next move, not unlike an analyst. He explains that D knew the police detectives would have assumed that the blackmailer would have concealed the letter in an elaborate hiding place, and thus hid it in plain sight. The deep unconscious appears on the surface of speech. The unconscious is like a very tall person walking with their feet at the bottom of the ocean while their mouth and speech remain above water.

Dupin says he had visited the minister at his hotel. In a cheap card rack hanging from a dirty ribbon, he saw a half-torn letter and recognized it as the letter of the story's title. Striking up a conversation with D about a subject in which the minister is interested, Dupin examined the letter more closely. It did not resemble the letter the prefect described so minutely; the writing was different, and it was sealed not with the "ducal arms" of the S family, but with D's personal or family monogram. A monogram is a written symbol made by overlapping or combining two or more letters, or graphemes, to form one symbol. In linguistics, a grapheme is the smallest functional unit of a writing system that corresponds with sounds (more accurately called phonemes). The prefect was lost in the details of the letter and ignored the real meaning. Also, in analysis there is no need to hear every word the analysand utters. Free association needs vacancy and emptiness.

Dupin noticed that the paper was worn by rubbing as if the stiff paper was first rolled one way and then another. Dupin concluded that D wrote a new address on the reverse of the stolen one, re-folded it the opposite way, and sealed it with his own seal.

Dupin left a snuff box behind as an excuse to return the next day. Resuming the same conversation, they had begun the previous day, D was startled by a gunshot in the street. While he went to investigate, Dupin switched D's letter for a duplicate.

Dupin explains that the gunshot distraction was arranged by him and that he left a duplicate letter to ensure his ability to leave the hotel without D suspecting his actions. If he had tried to seize it openly, Dupin surmises D might have had him killed. As both a political supporter of the queen and an old enemy of the minister [who had done an evil deed to Dupin in Vienna in the past], Dupin also hopes that D will try to use the power he no longer has, to his political downfall, and at the end be presented with a quotation from a play from Prosper Jolyot de Fébillon (A-treus and Thyestes) that implies Dupin was the real thief.

Dupin wonders what the Minister's reaction will be once he opens the fake letter, since once upon a time in Vienna, Austria, the Minister had offended him, and he had sworn at that time that he would not forget when D crossed paths with him (automaton or repetition compulsion because the offense will be compulsively repeated and revenged upon by Dupin). Now, Dupin has his quiet revenge of sorts, having written into the fake letter some lines that would suggest that it had been Dupin that had outsmarted him, or been one step ahead of D. These lines are apparently referenced in Dupin's own writing, saying that the Minister "is well acquainted with my manuscript". While implying that he outsmarts D, Dupin falls right into automaton's trap.

In the story, Lacan identifies three glances and three subjects (p. 10). The first subject or glance are the King and police that see nothing (the instant of seeing is not realized because the subject here is blind). The second subjects (Queen and Minister) see that the first subject sees nothing and believe to have covered or substituted what they are trying to hide. The third subject and glance are the Minister's and Dupin's who see that the second subjects have left the letter uncovered to whomever would seize it. In logical time, the different subjective positions refer to the birth of the blind subject as an impersonal subject. The impersonal subject designates a subjective position where different subjects, as variables, occupy certain positions in a structure according to their particular fantasies. This is the starting point of any psychical or mental formation.

Topologically, the unconscious appears outside or on the surface of the structure. At the end of the story, Dupin unconsciously moves from the position of the third subject to the position of the second subject by letting Minister D know his handwriting since he, like the Minister in his relationship to the Queen, is also depending upon "the robber's knowledge of the loser's knowledge of the robber". The story ends but the machine of repetitive automatism never stops. The robber's knowledge of the loser's knowledge of the robber refers to both D and the Queen, and D and Dupin, and the losers are both the Queen and the King. D knows that the Queen knows that D stole the letter for the purpose of blackmailing the Queen. In turn, D knows Dupin's manuscript as well as his writing.

The brief message Dupin wrote is an excerpt from the play A-*treus* and *Thyeste* by Frebillon, "A plan, if disastrous, or equally sinister, if it is not worthy of Atreus, is worthy of Thyestes". In Greek mythology this refers to two twin brothers, Thyestes and Atreus, who waged a bitter war of revenge against each other (automaton at work in myth and Greek tragedy). Under automaton, Dupin becomes another Minister D, and the two are twin brothers engaged in an imaginary rivalry. The moral of their story is that the process of revenge is ongoing, referring to the quotation. With this play, Dupin is implying that he takes revenge against Minister D by stealing the letter in the same way Minister D stole the letter from the Queen. Although much time has passed since Dupin had been offended by D in Vienna, he has now gotten revenge, and also managed to take 50,000 francs from the Prefect.

To conclude here is a basic outline of the metaphoric and substitutive elements of the structure and how subjects adopt actions by following the contours or acting in accordance with the structure. In reference to the symbolic structure the question can be asked: does the symbolic structure pre-exist and predicate the displacements of the letter, or is the symbolic structure created, established, or actualized by the displacements of the letter and the signifier?

1 A letter from the queen's lover has been stolen from her boudoir by the unscrupulous Minister D. D was in the room, saw the letter, and switched it for a letter of no importance. He has been blackmailing the queen.
2 The Prefect and Dupin know the content of the letter, but this is not disclosed. For Lacan the content is not important.
3 Dupin examined the letter more closely. It did not resemble the letter the prefect described so minutely; the writing was different, and it was sealed not with the "ducal arms" of the S family, but with D's family symbol. Although the letter is deformed in shape and bears a different name, it is still the letter. Dupin can recognize the letter because he is working on the technique of the signifier and its substitutions.
4 Dupin left a snuff box behind.
5 Dupin switched D's letter for a duplicate.
6 Minister opens fake letter.
7 The process of revenge about a sexual matter is ongoing, with the characters simply being substituted but replicating the same structure. Movement replicates the same structure in an overlapping manner. This understanding of the structure of the story is not unlike how an analyst, as tyche, reads a dream or the analysand's speech, producing an unexpected change in the automatism of the structure. In analyzing the story, Lacan exemplifies an analytic position. In this respect, the story does have a clinical significance that has been rarely touched upon in prior literature on the topic. This is despite the fact that Freud considered a literary background as fundamental for the formation of psychoanalysts. The function of reading or analyzing a narrative, as signifiers emerge in text or speech, and how this leads to the apperception of the signifying structure, seems to validate the hypothesis that the structure emerges or is revealed by the displacements of the letter and the signifier. The path and defiles of the signifier,

as they emerge in the experience of a personal analysis, can lead to different potential configurations of the symbolic structure. Here tyche at work in a present event precedes the automaton at work in the structure of repetition, while, at the same time, the structure of repetition remains open to the change afforded by the intervention of surprising factors that impinge upon the destiny of a subject.

Literary Significance and Criticism

This section begins with a brief overview of critical perspectives widely available, followed by an original in-depth discussion of the differences between Derrida's and Lacan's analysis of Poe's famous story and how these two views have galvanized and become central to the study of The Purloined Letter. Our position is that Derrida and Lacan are not that far apart and where they are it is because Derrida misunderstands Lacan and misunderstands the function of the Real and the Borromean knot of four of Lacan's later work.

Poe's story provoked a debate among literary theorists in the 1960s and 1970s. Lacan argued in Ecrits that the content of the queen's letter is irrelevant to the story and that the displacement of the signifier (the letter itself) is determined by the symbolic structure in which it exists and is displaced, first by the minister and then by Dupin. The minister and Dupin follow the displacement of the letter.

Other writers within literary criticism ironically gave a more typical psychoanalytic interpretation of the letter. Jacques Derrida, as examined below, responded to Lacan's reading in "Le Facteur de la vérité" ("The Purveyor of Truth"), pointing out what Lacan "missed" and suggesting that it is not that the letter lacks meaning, as Lacan claimed, but that Lacan made the lack the meaning. Unfortunately, Derrida and Deleuze do not understand or miss the structure of the lack and its relationship to the Real.

The truth, for Derrida, is that the letter is a castration of the King by the Queen, which Lacan cannot see or is blind to. In Derrida's view, both Poe's story and Andersen's (The Emperor has no clothes) feature a king whose virility and crown are imperiled, and who is saved by an individual who sees the obvious. The crown is saved from further embarrassment. Lacan's structuralist reading and Derrida's deconstructive reading provoked other psychoanalytic responses that suggested that the letter belonged all along to the Queen as a substitute for the phallus. Hull, following Michel Foucault, argued that "'The Purloined Letter' is a discourse on poetry's superiority over surveillance". For Foucault, surveillance by police agents is less important than the censoring function of metaphor and metonymy in language.

Derrida's Notion of "Phallologocentrism" vis-à-vis Lacanian Theory

Given the importance of Derrida's so-called post-structuralist thought, and the seriousness of his critique of Lacanian theory and Lacan's reading of Poe's text, we will dedicate this section to explore their differences in some detail.

First since Derrida was a philosopher who critiqued Lacan for having a non-rigorous grasp of philosophical thought, and of, like Heidegger, being stuck in ontological thought and essentialism, despite the corrections that Kantian thought brought upon Western thought. We will begin by discussing the philosophical underpinnings of Lacanian thought with reference to questions raised by Johnson and Hursh in their respective works on the subject. We do not intend to cover Lacan's overall comments on philosophy, which are extensive. Derrida uses Kant transcendental subject to philosophically critique Lacan of phallic monism, in agreement with Jung and Deleuze (1983), Derrida's Parisian philosophical contemporary.

Kant critiques ontology on the basis that it relies on synthetic a priori propositions that have no empirical support in the things in themselves. Concepts cannot yield knowledge of objects. Kant believed that in ontology there is no reference to sensory data although ontology does refer to the experiential realization of Being within the Sense function, or the Third jouissance of meaning, but beyond the senses.

> On Kant's account of the transcendental relation, then, one is obliged to take into account three rather than two terms: "phenomenal reality" as the constituted effect, and, working back to its transcendental conditions, the embrace between two irreducible poles: "the transcendental subject," described as an interpreting or synthesizing subject already equipped with certain sensory and cognitive powers, and an "object X," described as an existing materiality not created by us, to which we respond via receptive sensory systems.
>
> (Hursh, 2008, p. 20)

For Kant it is the cognitive faculties that organize the data coming from the senses and without them there would be no phenomena or a spatiotemporal manifold of objects rather than things. However, on the side of phenomena, Kant also believed that there was something in a phenomenon, which, despite not being a noumenon, is not exactly a grid of concepts organizing sensation either.

Existing materiality or "things in themselves" stimulate sensory systems, and while sensation in perception is interpreted according to language and symbolic systems, and although Kant did not believe that things in themselves can be cognized, Kant also proposes a hyletic substratum that lies somewhere in between the things in themselves, cognitive capabilities, and the symbolic and mental structures that determine them. Qualia, or the quality of sensations, are produced in between sensory signals arising from existing materiality, and perceptions that function as prevailing hypothesis about the world.

The hyletic substratum is the equivalent of das Ding in Lacan. Lacan speaks of the thing (chose) or the achose (the "no-thing") rather than the body or sache, the object in German. It is the word that makes and splits the thing and incorporates it in the process. When the word splits "the thing", das Ding is incorporated into the signifier. The word gives form to the thing, but also splits it in the process.

The objectivity of the thing is given by the signifier as an a priori category that constitutes an object of perception. The word splits the thing between the Real and the Symbolic. Half of the thing in itself remains in the Real, and outside the Symbolic, while the other half is incorporated into the signifier and the different levels of representation and the signifying chain.

Now how is the hyletic substratum related to the Real and das Ding? The hyle or the thing is not the same as the form of the word, and yet we don't know about it until it appears as a signifier, yet half of the hyle or truth of the thing remains outside the signifier. The hyle is the undetermined and the signifier represents the structure of determination. The hyle comes into existence through the signifier yet half of it "ex-sists" or remains outside symbolization. We could say it is analogous to the wave particle split or duality in quantum physics. Within the Real the thing is a wave, but in the Symbolic it manifests as a particle or signifying element.

The thing, as a signifier for the archaic mother (mater in Latin), remains the half of the thing that remains outside the signifier. The half that is incorporated into the signifier becomes the desire of the mother that is incorporated in the word or the Name of the Father. The desire of the mother is the half of the thing that is incorporated into the Symbolic through the NoF (Name of the Father). The other half remains outside and therefore can return as a thing that is disruptive of the Symbolic order.

However, jouissance is never entirely incorporated into the Symbolic order although it is also affected and effected by the signifier. The signifier casts and represents the shadow or hole of the absent thing that is not incorporated into the signifier. This hole is a vortex or a field of jouissance for the signifier; at the same time that jouissance is transformed by the structure of the signifier. The thing becomes an achose or a "nothing" by the intervention of the signifier, changing thereby the characteristics of the signifying field. For example, metaphor and metonymy may be inscribed with different forms of jouissance. It is metaphor that allows for the ring of the beyond the word to continue ringing past the word that evoked it, creating a possible communion between subjects.

However, Kant had more specific phenomena associated with the hyle such as sensations associated with sounds and images that are not yet the signifier. Lacan considered the relations of sounds, the phoneme, and the letter to the Real outside the signifier. He privileged homophony, or the similarity of sound, as a quality of the Real unconscious. Sound is more of a wave of subtle matter composed of less solid particles that create thereby a different form of field. Sound also represents the archaic world of objects before it was represented, and, in this respect, sound also represents images carried across space and converted into sounds, or images that one hears rather than sees. Is it possible to see sounds? Well, yes, we can see the images that are conveyed by sound waves that make letters that themselves make more images, when real objects materialize out of the signifier on a piece of a paper, or, out of the forms and edges of the letters themselves as seen in Arabic calligrams.

The hyle substratum however is a not a substance or an ether, a critique often made of ontology. The hyle is empty of essential nature until particles coalesce and survive to form matter. However, essential emptiness is a paradox because if emptiness is the essence, then essence is the same as no essence, ontology and anti-ontology being the same here in this example. There is no essence in emptiness and yet emptiness, like the Real, may represent a topological structure of dark matter within a dark field that undergirds the material structure of the observable universe, just as jouissance undergirds and supports the structure of the signifier. This would be the equivalent of hyle matter in Hebrew: Homer Hiyulih (חומר היולי).

Kant did not believe that there could be experience without conscious cognition or knowledge. We can think the things in themselves, but can we experience the things in themselves beyond conscious and unconscious thought, in non-thinking and non-knowing? What do we mean by knowledge in this case? Does knowing here mean knowing or experiencing a jouissance beyond the signifier? Is this the same as knowing how to distinguish colors or distinguishing sounds from visual images? This is not the same as knowing the content knowledge of various disciplines, for which there may be much disagreement.

True words and concepts always contain the ring of truth and jouissance that surpasses them. Therefore, Sophia or critical reason and Nous, as principal and principled forms of reason, are not without sensory experience of the thing, although such hyle of experience in the Real is not the same as the sensible material objects derived from the formal properties of reason and the signifier. Nous as the unmixed and pure form of reason gifts an experiential knowing of the One's own non-being, or a savoir based on the acceptance of a lack that energizes the words of those who speak.

On the one hand, the transcendental analytic or the categories of cognition are independent from experience because according to Kant (Hegel disagrees) an experience of the noumenon is not possible, and therefore any knowing of noumena represents a false cogito and knowledge. On the other hand, the analytic perspective critiques ontology for wanting a philosophical form of reason that is self-satisfied with concepts independent of any experience. The conclusion here is that only sense data represents experience while any experience outside logical and linguistic categories is systematically denied. What is missing here is the "ex-sistence" of any experience of jouissance, the drive, or desire outside symbolic coordinates.

The transcendental turn is not that different from the categorical imperative that considers any form of motivation other than duty as pathological. Of course, the sublimity of the categorical imperative is not without its foundations in experience and the sentiments as Hume and Confucius believed. To treat everyone as an end rather than as a means is precisely the logical articulation of the golden rule. The Other is not a means for the subject, because the object (a) is the heart of the experience of the subject and jouissance is the heart of the signifier. The transcendental turn paradoxically transcends experience and becomes profoundly at risk of a sense of obligation and compulsion where the truths or untruths of desire, or any form of kindness or existential care linked to the drive, are conceived, and repressed out of existence. This was one of Nietzsche's strongest objections to Kant's philosophy that militates against Nietszhe's work being reduced to Nazi ideology.

In psychoanalysis subjects report bodily experiences of jouissance triggered by a letter, or signifier, but where the significance or signified of the experience is not another signifier, but an experience of the body itself. This, however, does not mean that jouissance is something bodily rather than mental since satisfaction and pain are also mental constructs. Jouissance goes beyond the body mind duality. In the case of jouissance, mind means something beyond thinking and the signifier and points to the Real as a dimension of experience.

In the case of jouissance, the object of the drive is more in you rather than a subject or an objective object in the form of the X material object of knowledge in the external world as conceived by Kant. A false dichotomy is erected between objective knowledge derived from sense experience and the sensual knowledge of the senses that yields no reliable objective knowledge since the senses in the sense of the objects of desire only produce imaginary and idiosyncratic forms of knowledge/fiction.

For the senses to produce knowledge a filtering Sense function is required: f(k). However, symbolization and a symbolic order representing the laws and values of a culture, despite filtering the senses, also yields a reliable and valid knowledge regarding the fantasy in the treatment of mental disorders. Psychoanalysis would be a case example of a symbolic and objective form of subjectivity where the data is a patient's speech but not necessarily the quantification of their conscious social narratives according to themes or Likert scales.

In either case, whether in symbolic subjectivity or empirical data derived from the senses, the senses here no longer represent what the senses mean to an ordinary subject in the world. In everyday life the senses are linked to interests, needs, demands, and desires, but these senses are controlled, and not operative in the same way that sensory data works in science. Finally, the senses are not reliable sources of knowledge for phenomena that lie beyond our senses unless these are expanded by technology. Even then, beautiful Einstein had to rely on the Imagination to conceptualize what cannot be observed through the senses. Once the formulas emerged from his thought experiments, they could be confirmed by visual perception, but this could not have been accomplished the other way around. Imagination led to theory, and the theory led to theoretical observations, but the theory could not have been constructed without the imagination or the theory for the simple reason that you would have not known what to look for. It was the imagination and his theoretical mind that led him into the insights about the nature of light and gravity in nature, not the observational sense data that confirmed the former.

For Heidegger there is a primordial form of knowing that emerges inside a circle where a hidden empty positivity resides. This is consistent with Lacan's notion of unknown knowing, where one knows without knowing that one knows. "The One is the realization or knowing larger than the subject: The Unconscious in so far as it 'ex-sists'" (Lacan, 1971a, b, Seminar XIX, ...ou pire.). This is savoir without self-consciousness. Obviously, here the categories of knowledge represent savoir rather than knowledge (connaissance). Savoir is not the same as the conscious and a priori principles of formal reason, although it is not without logical articulation. As Hursh pointed out, truth cannot be consciously known too much or said for too long, without risking its deterioration and trivialization. Truth remains unconcealed but not unrevealed.

In addition, for savoir, knowledge functions more like a dark wave where each crest of the wave represents a moment of the contradiction but without an attempt to go back and synthesize the different contradictory moments. A wave of knowing simply keeps moving forward since the subquantum wave is what holds the different moments of the contradiction together, but each moment of the contradiction is independent of the other. A subquantum wave regulates the movement from Aletheia to Lethes and back to Aletheia, from remembering to forgetting. A subquantum field regulates which relative aspect of representational truth will be revealed in each crest of the wave that keeps moving knowing forward, but without synthesizing knowledge in each crest. A dark wave of jouissance, so to speak, is what contains the various moments of representational truth within the Real and beyond the Symbolic.

Derrida does not understand the Real or what Lacan means when he writes that the Real always returns to the same place. This place is not a particular object/signifier, but the very "no-thing" or jouissance that imbues knowledge and the signifier with the hands and feet of reality. It is the empty open hand that is most functional, not the hand that is already holding or grasping an object, or actually represents a closed fist. As we will show in the next chapter, for the later Lacan the proper place of the letter is the Real of jouissance rather than a phallic object or signifier. For the letter, significance or the signified can be in the Real, rather than in another signifier acting as a master signified.

The signifier itself has no self-identical place. The signifier is empty or missing from its place because the signifier cannot define itself: the signifier is always defined by the Other. The self-identical meaning of the signifier is outside the battery of signifiers and outside the symbolic because it precisely represents the intersection point between the Real and the Symbolic. The lack or emptiness of self-identity of the signifier, and the subject, coincides with the place of jouissance outside the signifier.

The meaning of the letter and its trajectory is the same as its destiny, north, orientation, or destination: meaning gives the signifier its trajectory, and the trajectory gives meaning to the signifier. For truth to have a destination or meaning in history it has to appear or be revealed on the side of semblance, representation, and fiction.

Derrida interprets the real as the proper place of symbolic castration where the letter always returns to. This is the only hold:

> It is, woman, a place unveiled as that of the lack of the penis, as the truth of the phallus, i. e., of castration. The truth of the Purloined Letter is the truth itself, its meaning is meaning, its law is law, the contract of truth with itself in the logos.
> (p. 60)

However, beyond the fiction of a master signifier that would serve as a transcendental guarantor of meaning, the hole of symbolic castration is more than simply a place of substitution for other signifiers. The hole is also the access point or index of the Real as something that lies outside the phallic order and the logos, and yet helps organize them at the same time.

Truth as the non-being of being is only understood by Derrida as veiled unveiled castration because Derrida has no understanding of the Real outside the text.

> As Lacan says elsewhere, the letter reverses to being (*la lettre revient a l'etre*); i.e., to that nothingness which is the openness (*l'ouverture*) as a hole between the woman's legs such is the proper place where the letter can be found, the words where meaning can be found, and where the minister believes it is the most protected, but we are in fact, in its very hiding place, it is the most utterly exposed.

The letter is a signifier. Derrida thinks the letter for Lacan is a phallic signifier of Lacan's early period. The letter more than a signifier is a non-phallic letter of jouissance as Lacan changed his teaching in Seminar XVIII. Here and now Lacan reduces emptiness to a vaginal hole, as the signifier of a lack that is identical to the phallus. 1 and -1, phi and -phi, have the same value in the Imaginary register. From this point of view Derrida is correct in saying that in this example the letter is reduced to a phallic object or signifier. Does the letter revert to emptiness and openness as a presence outside the signifier, or does the letter reverse to emptiness in the sense of a vaginal hole for the phallus, as if the vaginal hole represented the more generalized absence to which all words refer? The direct link to the object world has been lost, and instead language or other words stand in for the world, and for words, jouissance stands in the place where the direct link to the object world would have been before it was lost.

At this juncture we would have to ask whether for Derrida the phallus as a privileged object or master signifier is the same as its absence? In other words, whether the lack or the supremacy of the phallus and masculinity both amount to the same thing in the end? Is there no difference between a narcissistic egoic phallic parade of the imaginary phallus as a presence and the acceptance of symbolic castration and of the phallus as a signifier of a lack.

I guess Derrida's logic would reduce a black hole in physics to the dark opening between a woman's legs. Yeah sure, the dynamics of the galaxy in relation to the black hole at its center is all about fucking. Real non-being or emptiness is confused with the absence of being, itself conflated with the semblance or absence of an imaginary object a.

The letter returns to the body of the woman represented by the office of the minister, which is described as the body of a woman centered around the hole between the cheeks of the fireplace, and such is the proper place of the letter as the terminus, or end point, of a circular imaginary trajectory. "The letter returns to the sender who was not the signatory of the note but the place where it began to detach itself from its feminine possessor or inheritor The Queen" (p. 62). The NoF or King, is not the signatory of the note, instead the NoF is the signifying place that detaches the Queen from the meaning that her own genitals could become the signifier of the imaginary phallus.

The letter always returns to its Real place. Its address is the King, or the order of the law, but this address is a place of blindness, darkness, or not knowing where or how the law establishes its unconscious repressive effects, or guarantees the symbolic order of law, without subjects being aware of it. For Derrida's reductive reading of Lacan, the letter returning to its Real place always means the concept of the imaginary phallus or penis, or of the lack of an imaginary object.

However, a Real place also stands for the presence or experience of emptiness, das Ding, or the thing-in-itself. Socrates said to Alcibiades: there where you see an imaginary phallic object in me, I am nothing. The law is the law of the Real void, more than the law of the phallic signifier and prohibition. The law of the vacuum is the same as saying that the vacuum or the Real is without law because the law itself is void. The law of the void is that fresh tensions should be reduced to level zero, or at least to the lowest possible level that realizes a constancy within which the universe and subjects can exist. If the law of the void would be completely realized, as a true vacuum, then the universe itself and everything in it would instantaneously vanish, which in the Real, it does anyway.

Derrida also thinks that dissemination bears no relationship to the lack. Dissemination, as the act of spreading information widely, is covered under the metonymical characteristic of language, which, as we shall show in Chapter 3, does in fact have a relationship to the lack. Dissemination can also represent dissemination bias or the spreading of misinformation, or simply information in the sense of impersonal digital information rather than a subjective truth of desire represented by the signifier.

Derrida's dissemination bias, for example, has led to psychoanalysis being considered not only "phallologocentric" but also therapeutically ineffective. If one thing is constantly taken for another, this form of dissemination can prove to be dissembling of truth. Truth cannot be entirely said, and therefore the Real ring of truth is needed to ring beyond the signifier and the statement. Poetry and metaphor are suggestive of something beyond words that "lacks" signification and yet somehow functions within signification.

Derrida does not understand the lack, because he does not understand how the lack is related to metonymy, and how metonymy is related to dissemination. Derrida thinks that what guarantees the unity of the signifier, its point of stability, is the transcendental presence of the same signifier (the phallus) of signifiers underneath all the signified effects. Derrida confuses an ideal signifying order where signifiers have a fixed place, with the place of the Real as an emptiness or a hole that precisely permits and determines the movement of the signifier and its inability to define itself by itself. The flight or metonymy of the letter is due to it being senseless or is content having no meaning by itself other than as a form of jouissance.

Derrida's further criticism of Lacan, which Johnson's work underscores, may represent a straw man of Lacan and psychoanalysis in general. Derrida reduces Lacan's analysis of Poe's text to an analysis of subjective triads, as if these triads represented the unconscious signifying chains behind the narrative. This is the problem of discussing the theory of Oedipus, or triangles, outside the practice of analysis. It may seem relevant for the practice, but not as a thematic way to interpret the structure of a literary text, which is something that Lacan does not attempt to do anyway.

> The structure of the Purloined Letter cannot be reduced to a triangle unless the narrator is illuminated. The elimination of the narrator is a blatant and highly revealing result of the way psychoanalysis does violence to literature in order to find its own schemes. What psychoanalysis sees as a triangle is therefore really a quadrangle, and that forced side is the point from which literature problematizes the very possibility of a triangle. Therefore 3 = 4.
>
> (Hursh)

In addition, Johnson argues that "duality as such cannot be dismissed or simply absorbed into a triangle or structure. The Purloined Letter is traversed by an uncanny capacity for doubling and subdividing". Dual unity is not dismissed in psychoanalysis since it is an aspect of the dual fusion with the mother. The duality itself is not Imaginary since the Symbolic is made of binary components although not exclusively. The binary components themselves may function in non-binary modes or states (dual unity). The Third refers to the Other of the battery of signifiers and Names that pre-exist the subject. The Third is a Name and a word that symbolizes the subject and object of jouissance. Although in dual unity the infant is the subject and the mother the object, they do not become distinguished until they are named or symbolized. Once subject and object are named, they enter into the symbolic and psychical structure as discreet diacritical elements.

> The opposition between subjective and objective does not exist from the first. It is only constituted by the fact that thought has the ability to make present a second time something that was once perceived, by reproducing it in a representation, the outside object no longer having to be present.
>
> (Freud, 1925)

As shown in Chapter 3, doubling and subdividing are structural functions of metaphor and metonymy within the Third or the Other. However, there may be binary or alpha elements, as Bion calls them, that resist symbolization. Such elements function as imaginary translocation patterns to avoid entering into the triadic symbolization that is constitutive of metaphor and of the subject. Both in metaphor and in the subject, lack or emptiness occupies a central place. Instead, metonymy, as a distracting translocation pattern, represents the continuous movement to avoid the lack, of which Derrida's dissemination and critique of Lacan would be an example. Since metonymy does not sublate the signifier, metonymic representation is always tainted by lack in the attempt to avoid it. As has been shown in chaos theory in physics, movement and chaos are a sign of structure rather than lack of structure.

The fact that the structure has lack, or missing truth elements, fuels metonymic displacement within the structure or what Derrida calls dissemination.

Finally, another critique that Johnson mentions is that "The problem with this type of system, is that it cannot account for the possibility of sheer accident, irreversible loss, on unreappropriable residues, and infinite divisibility, which are in fact necessary and inevitable in the system's very elaboration". What the order of metaphor, sublation, and repression keeps "under surveillance and control is the uncanny itself, and the frantic anxiety which can be provoked, with no hope of reappropriation, enclosure, or truth".

Derrida misses how Lacan addresses the uncanny and the question of chance, particularly in the Suite that follows the Purloined Letter and that we will examine in a section down below in further detail. The Uncanny for Lacan is "the Thing" that represents something familiar appearing in an unfamiliar context, as well as something inanimate becoming animate or alive, as well as vice versa. Something appears where only absence should be expected, for example, an eye, or glaring gaze, inside a cut or vaginal hole.

Ignoring Lacan's ideas on the question of chance, Derrida presents chance as an alternative concept to the phallic signifier. Derrida contrasts the fixed Phallologocentrism of the Lacanian signifier with the chance aspects of the letter that Derrida thinks Lacan did not consider. For Derrida, the letter itself is presented in a series of coincidences and interconnection of cases and situations. For Derrida chance as writing, or writing as chance, is the "real subject of the tale". Writing, chance events, and coincidences go together.

Derrida says that chance, surprise, or coincidence is the real subject of a tale, implying the subject and the reader as holders of Real jouissance, and the meaning or logical structure embedded in a story. Meaning or the signifier is supposed to bring forth the experience of the author, in the experience of the reader, as the holder of the chance epiphanies of the author. Structure is preceded and followed by chance events.

Accident represents the coincidence of the word. A narrative only appears to be made up of random observations. An observer perceives the imaginary impregnations that pose as substitutes or alternatives for the structural elements that are otherwise known to the theory. The analyst is fond of the enigmas, conundrums, and hieroglyphics that appear in the interstices between the structural elements, and the imaginary impregnations that surround them. It is the word or the signifier that anticipates the coincidences for the subject within the net of language. Over the course of a subject's life, the itinerary of the signifier takes the subject to this or that mis/encounter with various forms of meaning and experience.

Lacan's Theoretical Itinerary

> p. 6. My research has led me to the realization that repetition automatism has its basis in what I have called the insistence of the signifying chain. I have isolated

> this notion as a correlate of the "ex-sistence" in which we must necessarily locate the subject of the unconscious, if we are to take Freud's discovery seriously.

Here it is interesting to see how Lacan uses a term coined by Heidegger (ek-sistence). Lacan uses the term "ex-sistence" to refer to the ego being decentered by the repetition compulsion, the Ucs. signifying chain, and the subject of the unconscious that occupies an eccentric place relative to the conscious ego. The insistence of automaton produces the subject of the unconscious which is eccentric to the ego.

Later in his work Lacan will refer to "ex-sistence" as jouissance and what is outside the signifier, signaling a move from the Symbolic to the Real. Jouissance is eccentric to the subject, in the same way that the subject is eccentric to the ego. Not only does the signifier replace or stand in for conscious ego-knowledge (connaissance), but jouissance in the Real is also outside the signifier yet organizes its internal structure.

Since many of you may not know the meaning of the word and concept of jouissance we will define it for you. Jouissance has not been translated in English because enjoyment in English or original happiness in Chinese do not contain the meaning of suffering that is also associated with jouissance. In fact, despite what people say, in French the word also means pleasure or the little death of orgasm, but this does not imply suffering. Jouissance is a concept more than a word.

Jouissance refers to increases of tension, both pleasant and unpleasant, that violate, according to Lacan, the pleasure principle that aims at lowering tensions. Jouissance can represent satisfaction or suffering, something pleasant or unpleasant. The signifier and desire, operating according to the pleasure principle, want to lower the tensions associated with jouissance. However, this was only the early conception of jouissance in Lacan as inconvenient and destructive. The signifier and the Symbolic stop this inconvenient jouissance so that a desire can be reached that is compatible with the Law, at the same time that this desire is linked to the experience of phallic jouissance, or what is enjoyable and painful about phallic jouissance and sexuality.

Finally, phallic jouissance also fails to represent a form of satisfaction since it is always a question of who is or is not, has or has not the phallus. The symbolic phallus as an absence and symbolic castration function as a portal for the satisfaction associated with the Third jouissance. The Third jouissance has three forms that function outside the Symbolic and the phallic order. The three are feminine jouissance, the jouissance of the mystic, and the jouissance of meaning.

> Page 11. I am, of course, aware of the importance of imaginary impregnations in the "partializations" of the symbolic alternative that give the signifying chain its appearance. 3rd paragraph. Page 11

The imaginary impregnations can be seen in the case of the "Rat Man". This was the nickname given by Sigmund Freud to a patient whose "case history" was published as "Notes Upon a Case of Obsessional Neurosis" (1909). The nickname derives from the fact that among the patient's many compulsions was an obsession with nightmarish fantasies about rats. In the case of the Rat man Freud points out how names and linguistic signifiers, as a signifying chain, can be used to make connections between Ucs. thoughts (fantasies or memories) and symptoms (the thoughts the Rat man had about the cousin and the obsession). The fantasies and the symptoms represent the imaginary impregnations on the signifying chain.

Imaginary signifiers in the symptoms and fantasies have to be used as the symbolic alternatives to reveal the signifying chain. In other words, the jouissance in the symptom has to be affected not by interpretation in the sense of an explanation, but by releasing the jouissance contained within the letters and the signifying chain, transforming it in the process. The structure is always a melodrama, but the characters change. In the rat man, the imaginary signifier fat is associated with the name Dick that means fat in German but also to the Name of his competitor for the love of a lady for whom he wants to make himself thinner (another imaginary impregnation).

> p. 15 Thus, when we are open to hearing the way in which Martin Heidegger uncovers for us in the Greek word alethes the play of truth, we merely rediscover a secret to which truth has always initiated her lovers, and through which they have learned that it is in hiding that she offers herself to them most truly, the signifier – you are perhaps beginning to catch my drift – materializes the instance of death.

In his work, Heidegger (1943) tries out different approaches to the question of truth. Aletheia or aléthes, for example, refers to two things: both aléthes and léthes, truth and concealing or forgetting. "In every entry of being into its habitation in words, there's a margin of forgetting, a lethe complementary to every aletheia" (Lacan, 1953–1954, p. 192). When truth enters into words, the other half of truth in the Real of jouissance is forgotten. But this is the same as saying that when the subject is represented by the signifier, the subject as a jouissance outside the signifier is forgotten and falls into a Real dimension of truth where the subject is represented by a trace of jouissance. If the subject attempts to cling on to the signifier as a form of identity, then the identification with the imaginary phallic signifier will only fixate the subject to miserliness and hatred, as Lacan says.

> But as for the letter itself, it can be taken in many ways, in the sense of the metonymic polyvalence of the signifier: whether we take the letter in the sense of a typographical element, of an epistle, or of what constitutes a man of letters, we commonly say that what people say must be understood a la lettre (to the letter or literally), that a letter is being held for you at the post office, that cannot even be designated late mail.
>
> (p. 17)

> For the signifier is a unique unit of being which, by its very nature, is the symbol of but an absence. This is why we cannot say of the Purloined Letter that, like other objects, it must be or not be somewhere but rather that, unlike them, it will be and will not be where it is wherever it goes.
>
> p. 17. Last paragraph. "That it will not be in its place" can literally [to the letter] only be said of something that can change places – that is, of the Symbolic. For the real, whatever upheaval we subject it to, is always and in every case in its place; it carries its place stuck to the sole of its shoe, there being nothing that can exile it from it.

The use of the future tense implies the logical time that there will be a retroactive effect in the future: the letter "will not be" where it goes because the future points repetitively to the past. During this period of his work the real is interchangeable with the ground of environmental or external social reality. However, he already hints at the later notions that the Real is something that always stays the same as an absolute difference and can be found everywhere. We capitalize the Real to disambiguate the concept of the Real from the social or external reality (Freud's reality principle).

During this period of his work, Lacan understood the letter on the model of the phoneme as a building block of the symbolic order and the structure of language. During his later period, the letter is understood more in terms of homophony or the similarity between sounds, and the relationship between the letter and the Real, more than in terms of the relationship between the letter and the Symbolic. Finally, where the signifier "will be and will not be" is also a description of the topological trajectory of the signifiers. In the case of metonymy and displacement the signifier is changing places, while in the case of metaphor and jouissance, the subject always returns to the same place, while the signifying structure remains the same because it is the same syntax that underlines the structure of automaton.

A Letter is a typographical element, and a metaphor for a person of letters or an intellectual. At a literal level of meaning, a postal letter is not an object that may or may not be somewhere, because as a signifier it will always be and not be somewhere for structural reasons. A letter is also a litter in the sense of how a letter can impregnate a cat or a human, and a litter also represents a recyclable waste product such as the objet a. The symbolic is what changes the places for the objet a, from the Imaginary to the Real. The Real instead always stays in the same place. The Real cannot be fully translated into language or the Symbolic, and, therefore, cannot be metonymically displaced, but its jouissance is subject to metamorphosis and transformations.

Jouissance and the signifier are of different orders (Real and Symbolic) but are not incompatible. Jouissance and the signifier are incommensurable in the sense that there is no metalanguage that would resolve/reduce/translate them to a common language or standard, but they are compatible in the sense that they interpenetrate: there are words of jouissance (lalangue) and jouissance within words.

Jouissance within words is an implicit quality of speech and of the word well said that sustains and reveals the "ex-sistence" of the word, and how the word is organized outside the symbolic order.

When subjects think that they are using the letter (through imaginary impregnations), this is actually an instance of the letter determining the meaning of their actions and their consequences. By coming into the letter's possession – an admirable ambiguous bit of language – its meaning possesses them. (When subjects think they possess their objects of desire, their objects of desire possess them.) Such is the signifier's answer, beyond all significations: "You believe you are taking action when I am the one making you stir at the bidding of the bonds with which I weave your desires".

Yin and Yang

> For in playing the game of the one who hides, Dupin is obliged to don the role of the Queen, including even the attributes of woman and shadow, so propitious for the act of concealment. I do not mean to reduce the veteran couple of Yin and Yang to the primal opposition of dark and light. For their precise handling involves what is blinding in a flash of light, no less than the shimmering that shadows exploit in order not to release their prey.
>
> (p. 22)

Lacan refers to how Dupin is obliged to function as woman and shadow in order to conceal his investigation. This is a question of concealment in exposition and exposition in concealment. Compare this statement with the Cantongqi poem by Chan (Zen in Japan and Korea) teacher Shito Chichin from the eighth century in China.

Within light there is darkness, but do not be caught by that darkness,

Within darkness there is light, but do not be blinded by that light or see it as light.

Light and darkness are a pair, like the foot before and the foot behind, in walking.

Within the light of a phenomenal event lies a deep structure of determination or automaton, but do not be caught by the dark structure in which the event is embedded. Illumination in perception includes the apperception of the structure that makes the event intelligible, while at the same time the energy of the event can renew or change the underlying structure of determination.

If the subject is not blinded by the light within darkness, and the dark is kept dark, then in analysis, this is the level of interpretation that goes from the unknown to the unknown. In a clinical example an analysand was ambivalent about having two sessions a week but could not give a reason. In the next session he began by saying that my waiting room was "too weak". In response, I offered the mentioned interpretation: "Two a week is too weak". Two a week is left unexplained, and so is the "too weak" referring to the waiting room. But in bringing the two together through an enigmatic interpretation, a signifying effect is produced in the Real jouissance of the subject "ex-sisting" in between signifiers and speech acts.

Jouissance can be darkness or suffering, or jouissance can represent a satisfying form of bliss and realization. In addition, suffering can be represented as light and not only darkness, or as the darkness within the light; and bliss and realization can be represented as dark forms of unknown knowing without self-consciousness. The example of the blind seer, or the wisdom of the blind, would be a case in point. The inconvenience of jouissance must be passed over or transformed by not clinging to the light, or the darkness within the light. On the other hand, darkness is a form of "endarkment", or an intense beam of darkness present within the light. Such light within darkness needs to be kept in the dark and realized as the forms of the world: the light in speech, and the light packages that thanks to the Borromean knot are perceived as the forms of the world. The object is not an image, but as the "thing" or "no-thing", the object is a form of jouissance outside the signifier.

Here the sign and being, marvelously disjoint, reveal which one wins out when they are opposed. A man who is brave enough to scorn a woman for her dreaded ire suffers the curse of the sign or letter that he has taken from her. The missing letter, in turn, also causes the Queen to undergo a metamorphosis.

Within the light of the surface where the Minister finds the letter, and the light in which the investigation takes place, there is the darkness of the Queen's actions and non-actions and her reputation. The Minister, captured by this darkness, took the position of the feminine by taking the same action and non-action of the queen in playing the game with the prefect as the Queen did with the King. This is also why Lacan says both the King and the prefect take the position of the first subject. Making a metamorphosis of the letter and then pretending to be careless by laying bare there an achievement of meticulous effort, on the obvious place, is really a feminine position.

Within darkness the Queen suffers the curse of the visible sign that has gone missing. The letter causes the Queen to undergo a silent metamorphosis. Here undergoing a metamorphosis within her subjectivity means that by receiving the letter and losing it, the queen becomes dangerous to the King by breaking their marriage vows and risking the break-up of their contract, and the country's safety thereby.

In reference to this Lacan writes:

> For this sign is clearly that of woman, because she brings out her very being therein by founding it outside the law, which ever contains her – due to the effect of origins – in a position as signifier, nay, as fetish. In order to be worthy of the power of this sign, she need but remain immobile in its shadow, managing thereby, moreover, like the Queen, to simulate mastery of nonaction that the Minister's "lynx eye" alone was able to see through.

Then on p. 23 we read:

> The letter's power departs when used, we perceive that this remark concerns only its use for ends of power – and simultaneously that the Minister will be

> forced to use it in this way…For it is clear that while the Minister will be forced to make use of the letter in a non-significant way, its use for ends of power can only be potential, since it cannot become actual [passer a l'acte] without immediately vanishing.

A woman gives out a sign that brings out her very Being that is established outside the signifier and the Law. The letter cannot be used as a means for power without the letter vanishing as a consequence. Whenever power is actualized or acted out, it vanishes. The imaginary phallus does not ultimately exist, and the signifier is a signifier of a lack, so the imaginary phallus cannot be used as a positive sign of power or privilege without it turning into a pure signifier of the lack in the Other. Power is the power of the lack, of the missing signifier, of the emptiness above the crown of power, of the power of the human spirit rather than the power of might, domination, or privilege. Thus, Lacan says that the letter exists as a means of power only through the final summons of the pure signifier.

> The audacious creature is, of course, reduced here to the state of imbecilic blindness in which man finds himself in relation to the wall-like letters that dictate his destiny.
>
> (p. 29)

Yes, no doubt, for if "any point requiring reflection", as Dupin states at the start, is examined "to better purpose in the dark (imbecile blindness)", we may now easily read its solution in broad daylight because the letters have written the destiny of the subject on the wall. This is a topological truth; the inside is outside, and the unconscious depth is on the surface. Secret thoughts, as well as analysis and its treatment effect, are better examined in private although the consequence of this process will be revealed in broad daylight and everyday situations.

This is why what the Purloined Letter means the letter "en souffrance", or the missing or lost letter that has not arrived, means that a letter always arrives at its destination through topological detours. The only letter that does not arrive is the one that has not been written. The Queen happily received a private and secret romantic or sexual letter, which then became a very public letter, and yet the King never found out although everything around him was affected by it. For the sake of the nation, the reputation of the King was protected at all costs. Nowadays the opposite may be true in the West, in a self-destructive and masochistic act any mistake or flaw of the leader must be compulsively revealed despite the cost to the nation. Lacan translates the Shakespearian King into the "nothing" of the phallus, as the lack in the Other.

> Hamlet: The body is with the King, but the King is not with the body. The King is a thing – Guildestern: A "thing", my lord? Hamlet: Of nothing …
>
> (H, IV-ii, 27–30)

When the King died, and died of treachery, the King became a signifier of nothing. The great "Thing" is nothing in this case. As the monosyllable word, it can also be the sound and sound only. But the King not only represents a miserable "cornuto" or "cockhold", the "nothing". The King also represents the emptiness of the spirit of the nation.

The Suite

The Suite that follows the Purloined Letter includes a detailed incursion into binary logic and computer programming. The relation between letters and numbers is complex. On the one hand, letters are meant to be read while numbers are used to perform arithmetical operations and functions. On the other hand, letters as variables can be used to perform arithmetical operations, and numbers can be read symbolically and metaphorically (think of the number 1 for example, as in the phrase: "you are the 1"). Letters and numbers both have an effect outside meaning or can be senseless units that must be combined to generate meaning within a system.

The two features of a jouissance effect outside meaning, and how letters are senseless units of meaning that combine to produce meaning inside a signifying system or structure, are the components of a GEB number system in Hofstadter's (1979) work.

Lacan's formulation of the Symbolic as a formal language incorporates formal logic, Boolean logic, and the binary logic invented by Leibniz and prevailing in the field of computer programming, cybernetics, and cognitive psychology. Lacan's interest in binary logic responds to the attempt to understand and develop Freud's idea that the unconscious determines the conscious ego. He wanted to figure out how a formal language determines the subject even if it is the "active" subject that engages such a language. Like in all logic and mathematics, problems and equations require repeated practice and exercises. This is precisely what Lacan attempts to do in the "Suite" following the text on The Purloined Letter. In The Purloined Letter, repetition is motivated by the displacement of the letter, while the displacement of the letter is actually the reappearance of the letter in different places. This reappearance corresponds to the repeated exercises of The Suite. In addition, there is a loss involved in every repetition.

Such efforts take Lacan outside the parameters used by Freud to define the unconscious. Even though Freud was well aware of how the unconscious worked within language (in jokes, dreams, and everyday life), Freud believed that images and not words prevailed in the unconscious. It was Lacan's contribution to give an account of the signifying chain operating within the unconscious. However, in 1955 he had not yet developed the concept of the signifying chain with the aid of the graph of desire or the concept of the Real in its two periods.

One of the important merits of Lacan's text is how he links Freud's clinical and phenomenological observation of the Fort-Da game in a child, with an exposition of the Even or Odd (Head or Tails) game as it appeared in The Purloined Letter. Both serve as examples of how the symbolic order is the world of the machine.

Lacan also plays upon the pun of Odd as both an odd number and the queer or bizarre feature of the itinerary and defiles of the signifier. This oddity is signaled by the letter as leading the movement of signifiers and as designating the syntax's failure (i.e., slips of the tongue) manifesting itself within the symbolic order. As we see, contrary to what Derrida believed, the ambiguous and equivocal use of the signifier is not based on a transcendental phallic meaning, but on the chance factors associated with automaton and Tyche.

As the f(O)rt d(A) example or observation constitutes an empirical/structural moment of psychoanalytic developmental theory, the Even/Odd game represents a foundation for probability theory. The result of the combination amounts to an informal proof of how automaton, as a supposed form of chance, or randomness, represents an actual form of causal determination. The probability of a win or a loss is already determined by the structure and articulation between win and loss, head or tails, + or −. This form of chance or randomness is how the Real first appears to Lacan. For Lacan of this period, the Real means the syntax of automaton which makes automaton appear as randomness.

Tyché and Automaton

The early Real in Lacan is ominous, painful, awful, hazardous, accidental, and is often not differentiated from the concept of external reality in general or the two are used interchangeably. The second Real is more like tyché, a true hole that generates consonance and concord, or is benevolent and auspicious. This view coincides with tyché as the Greek goddess of Fortune as something surprising and undetermined at the heart of the structure of determination, the point where structure vanishes or does not exist. Once the structure of determination and symbolic effectiveness is realized by a subject, the entire structure disappears, or temporarily vanishes from existence, and the subject withdraws from its circuit. Confucius said that a sage should occupy positions of administration and governance, but then withdraw as soon as possible to avoid imaginary group power effects. Tyche represents the necessary vanishing of the signifier and power, lest they fall in the hands of the ego and automaton which they will use for destructive purposes. If the imaginary ego clings to the signifier, then automaton will transform the power of the signifier into human dramas or fateful tragedies filled with suffering, jealousy, envy, and hatred between people.

Automaton and Tyché are the two forms of chance that Aristotle considered. In the Suite or Exercises, the two are not clearly differentiated and both are subsumed under the principle of the repetition compulsion. "What are you, figure of the dice I roll in your chance encounter (tyché) with my fortune?". The chance encounter in this case refers to a point of fortune rather than the repetition of a conflict or a trauma. It is important to "remember" that in Beyond the Pleasure Principle, Freud (1920) pointed out that repetition in trauma or the return to the place of trauma is not only a daemon of repetition, but also an attempt at catharsis, healing, and repetition with a difference that makes all the difference. Within the symbolic structure there are two kinds of repetition: one is automaton seemingly as random chance but actually determined. The other one is the repetition designated by the Collatz sequence; it repeats but the destination is not always known. Tyche is the repetitive encountering of both forms of the Real in the practice but the where and when is unknown. Using Collatz number, we can describe Tyche and how the One can be achieved or not achieved, and what is described as decidable or not.

Although we know that as a therapeutic practice, psychoanalysis makes a necessary and moderate use of chance, luck, and opportunity or surprise, does Tyche appear in Poe's or Lacan's text on the Purloined Letter? Clearly, Poe's text is overdetermined by automaton as a false form of chance, but does Tyche play any part in the text? Are automaton and Tyche logically connected? In Lacan's analysis of the text, the itinerary of the signifiers is articulated by automaton, but within automaton, as a form of actual psychical causality, there lies the gap where Tyché can appear. Automaton brings us once again to the repetitive scene, while Tyché, in the verbalizing process of analysis, as an epiphany, or as a sudden encounter/mis-encounter with the Real, breaks up the chain of automaton, and culls the living flower of desire.

The Lacanian concept of the Real eludes and disconcerts because it is situated in a dimension beyond formal logic/binary language and the senses and yet it is intrinsically "bound up" with language and the senses. Lacan links the Real to the concept of Tyché in Aristotle. Aristotle (350 BCE/2002) distinguished between causality and chance as an accidental form of causality. In the Physics, Aristotle distinguishes between two modes or types of causality: causality proper (four causes) and two kinds of chance. The two kinds of chance are automaton and Tyché. It is important to distinguish between the two types of causality (causality proper and chance) and the two types of chance because these are often confused. In fact, Lacan also refers to Tyché as a form of causality instead of as a form of accidental causality. In the Ecrits, the Real is the syntax of automaton. Tyche instead is the encounter or mis-encounter with the Real as a true form of chance.

More recently, after Aristotle, Hume (1748, Of Probability) distinguished between causality and probability. Due to our ignorance or the limitations of our cognitive and perceptual functions we miss many small, numerous, or complex forms of causality. At some point complexity renders prediction impossible. From this perspective, the most we can know is various degrees of probability that certain events may be causally related to one another.

Chance is an everyday word used when speaking about an event taking place while probability is a precise measurement of that chance. In the roll of the dice, each of the six numbers/sides of a dice has a 1/6 chance of manifesting. Probability is a special branch of mathematics that helps people decide the percentage of likelihood of an event taking place (according to a large number of computer runs or calculations).

For Aristotle (Physics) there were two forms of chance or accidental/spontaneous/ random causality: Tyché and automaton. Of the two only Tyché is truly spontaneous or Real. Automaton appears random because it disrupts predictable social behavior derived from social norms but is determined by very precise signifying chains of conscious or unconscious causality. Automaton is the disruptive psychical causality associated with the Freudian Unconscious while Tyché is the type of chance linked to the Lacanian Real unconscious.

Automaton is more characteristic of nature and "unreasoning agents" as in the example of animal instincts. Here the connection between unconscious psychical causality, nature, and instinct cannot fail to be made. Automaton as unconscious determination is also linked to chance and its derivation from the Latin cadere – to fall, and to fall away from the norm and toward decadence. Games of chance are also associated with decadence and with leaning or decline rather than being upright.

For Lacan the Real is beyond and behind automaton and can be linked to accidental events that have an effect on a subject's destiny (Tyche) and this is to be distinguished from fate that represents a fall as in the case of Oedipus who ended up killing his father, and marrying his mother, despite his otherwise preconscious and socially acceptable intentions.

Tyche is undetermined, surprising, and accidental, but responds to automaton and repetition. Tyche as the Real destiny of the subject always brings the subject back to the same place. But this is a different form of repetition. Fateful automaton is always displacing, and yet this form of change is nothing new since it simply replicates a structure that turns around a hole of turbulence, disturbing forms of jouissance, and repressed or missing signifiers. Thus, there are two forms of repetition: destructive and constructive, or demon and daimon. Tyche is a form of daimon. Automaton is a form of mental automatism, the most extreme form of which is the clanging associations observed in acute psychoses.

But automaton could also be any bad old habit or repeated mistake. Tyche responds more to virtuous repetition whereby by performing a good habit the subject becomes prone to enlightening accidents of discovery and creation. It is like the metaphor of the good and bad dummy, puppet, Golem, robot, wooden man, and stone woman. A subject can act without self-consciousness and let the signifier "enlighten" the subject, or the subject can simply be a subjected wooden object to be used by another subject and their desire. The first is Tyche; the second is automaton.

Some authors confuse automaton with causality proper. This is not accidental (pardon the pun) given that automaton is a type of chance that only appears to be arbitrary or contingent. In fact, automaton is the result of structural and unconscious unintended consequences. For example, a person wanted to say one thing and instead said the opposite. Here chance in the sense of change only appears to be something new or spontaneous. Automaton is the permutation of pre-determined structural factors. Change or chance here does not escape determinism. This is particularly true of unconscious psychical causality and the repetition of trauma and suffering, whether in pain or pleasure, in desiring the desires of others or repeating their painful mistakes.

Perhaps the key to the text, in this respect, is that automaton is not allowed to reach a point of maximum destructiveness where the hostile intentions of the characters in the structure of the story could lead to the annihilation of the individual characters and the entire structure of the nation as a system of symbolic exchange. D's repetition is controlled by Dupin as a chance element that both repeats and transforms the jouissance contained within the structure. D represents only automaton and repetition while Dupin represents automaton but also the possibility of Tyche with the caveat that Dupin be furthered transformed into an analyst.

In the Purloined Letter, with the example of Dupin, Lacan wants to show how stubborn repetition can be upon the subject. In Lacan's analysis, Dupin is the idealized amateur detective because he is also prey to automaton. And his narcissistic way of explaining the process of finding the letter is determined by automaton. In a certain sense, Dupin can be taken as the allegorical image of the analyst who fails when stuck in the SsS (Subject Supposed to Know) position of being the subject supposed to know.

> There's a double benefit to be gained by identifying Dupin with the psychoanalyst from the beginning: first, the lucidity of he who can see what no one else can: the place of the thing, between the legs; second, the possibility in creating the impression that Dupin continues to be a participant (and how), and in maintaining the identification of Dupin with the psychoanalyst, of denouncing the naivete of the community of endless, of saying: you psychoanalysts, you delude yourselves at the very moment when, like Dupin you think you are the Masters. (p. 72)

In the end Dupin is considered to have broken off his temporary identification with the minister and remains the only one who all of the sudden and surprisingly sees everything that is taking place within the structure. Tyché is the more distinctly human type of chance which, on the one hand, represents the possibility of something truly arbitrary, contingent, as well as new, but can also be linked to what Aristotle called luck or virtue in the sphere of ethical actions.

Although the results/effects of moral choice appear undetermined until a choice is made, the only thing undetermined is the emptiness or the yet undefined nature of the choice itself. The structure and arc of possible choices, and what the consequences may be, are pre-determined. However, depending on the choice the results may vary and may lead to different permutations of the structure. Human nature is undetermined or unfixed until a choice is made and the outcomes of our choices return in the various forms of causality including automaton.

The unary trace, like a footprint in the sand, or a mark on a tree, is simply an instance not in the sense of agency, but in the sense of a moment in time or a vanishing point instant. A trace is a mark or a notch that can be effaced and once erased it remains as a potential unit that is always self-same, meaning that other than quantity or number of times, there are no differences produced in the iterations of the same thing. Natural numbers and the alphabet are systems composed of diacritical signs and signifiers.

The signifier has even less material existence than the trace but is preserved as a system of written signs in the mind of the subject and the culture although not always in explicit manner. Silence or the absence of speech and writing is always an option. Thus, Lacan will say that the trace is effaced while the signifier is either repressed or abandoned but not unsignified or unmarked, due to its relations to other signifiers. What remains unmarked within the signifier itself is its inability to signify itself by itself.

In the story, the Queen is the victim of her imaginary desires and fantasies that are not represented in the story, but also of the social symbolic censorship that is also not explicitly stated in the story. D is the allegory of the subject of automaton, while Dupin is the allegory of the analyst of automaton. The three of them remind us that the imaginary phallus does not exist, and that once the subject is captured by its logic, an infinite imaginary impersonation of both the subject and the other may appear in a story to represent both the pre-subject (as the mother's imaginary phallus) and the inexistant imaginary phallus.

In a Lacanian sense, Poe exhibits how the subject is constructed within the symbolic and with the ego's own imaginary input. However, with a Lacanian reading of the story, Dupin and his way of interacting with the structure of the story can be understood as an allegory of a failed analysis. But through this interpretation, when the analyst lets go of the position of being the subject supposed to know, this can also be understood as a Tyche moment in any analysis that frees the signifier to have a curative effect upon the Real of a bodily jouissance outside the automaton represented by the signifying structure.

The Letter and the Signifier

In this section we want to consider the function of the letter as an index of jouissance (both pathological and curative) introduced into a text. The function of the letter as an index of jouissance is only implicitly present in the Ecrits and will not manifest until Lacan's (1970–1971) Seminar XVIII "On a Discourse that might not be a Semblance". The same is true for jouissance. The term only appears in a preliminary form in Lacan's text on Poe. The later notion of jouissance (seminar XX and XXIII) appears in the Ecrits in the paper on the subversion of the subject and the dialectic of desire but the Third jouissance had not yet been differentiated from the first two forms of jouissance.

In Lacan's later work the letter precipitates an influx and outpouring and evacuation of jouissance. Jouissance animates and both disrupts and brings cohesion to the signifying structure. This function of the letter is not yet present in the Ecrits paper dedicated to the instance of the Letter in the Unconscious. The Unconscious in the Ecrits is the repressed Freudian unconscious, while the unconscious of jouissance is the Real unconscious. The signifier and the symbolic order are organized by S_1–S_2 relations that Lacan will later on define as a semblance, while the letter in relationship to jouissance, I argue, is organized by an S_1–S_0 relation.

In the Ecrits Lacan focuses mainly on the letter's function of representing a hole or something missing within the symbolic order. Its main function is to be the material support, texture, and localized structure of the signifier. Words are made of various combinations of letters that originally represented something else. Because the letter is a missing letter, every letter erases itself in composing a word and becomes symbolized by being sound differentials. In this construction, when the letter is taken as a distinguishing structure rather than as letter, the letter becomes a functional element. But this is only a camouflage in function because the letter is never only functional. The letter is both a site of jouissance and the place where repression works most effectively. By losing itself as a simple differential, by being solely a sound, a shape, its own meaning becomes a hole of jouissance. Only the third jouissance gives a Real position to the subject.

Regarding the hole of jouissance, Lacan spoke of a true hole and a false hole. The Freudian unconscious is a false hole in the sense that in the hole lies a repressed signifier of the objet a, while in the true hole the objet a gains access to the Real beyond the signifier. A hole or gap is false because, like automaton, it is not without cause. Now when the gap is within the acausal, then this is a true hole of "undetermination" and indetermination.

We said above that the inexistence of the imaginary phallus, and of the imaginary ego (other than as a matheme or logical concept), as a gap or lack within the symbolic structure, points to how a symbolic structure represents the object of the drive, its prohibition, and the subject itself, through a series of displaced and inverted narratives and stories. The signifier functions as a semblance when the signifier is used to close the hole represented by the inexistence of the ego and the imaginary phallus.

In the Ecrits Lacan says that the letter cannot be used as a means for power without the letter vanishing as a consequence. This definition of power represents power as the power of domination and the reification of this power, not the power of symbolization itself. The power of metaphor and signification has already replaced whatever minor or major role the master's imaginary ego had to play in its production. Whenever power is turned into domination or acted out, sooner or later, it vanishes. The imaginary phallus does not ultimately exist, and the signifier is a signifier of a lack, and thus the imaginary phallus cannot be used as a positive sign of power or privilege without it turning into a pure signifier of the lack in the Other within the structure.

In his seminar "On a Discourse that might not be a Semblance" Lacan (1971) worked on two related themes: first, that the signifier/representation is nothing more than a semblance (1/13/71-I 9) and, second, that the signifier is Symbolic while the letter is Real (12/5/71-p.VII 14). With the latter distinction Lacan reflects on the possible existence of a discourse based on the letter and its relationship to the littoral or a region lying along the shore of a lake or sea (lituraterre instead of literature). The semblant points to the intersection between the Symbolic and the Imaginary, whereas the letter lies between the Symbolic and the Real. The whole point of rethinking the letter in the light of the Real of jouissance is to show how the psyche, psychoanalysis, and the Borromean knot cannot be limited to the Symbolic and the Imaginary. In addition, the Real cannot be limited to Lacan's first conception of the Real as automaton.

Semblance or "the semblant" is a word/concept that has two different yet related meanings. The first refers to the classical distinction between appearance and reality. The second acceptation refers to the face or countenance. Appearance and face are also related through the concept of the mask and the Jungian concept of the persona that represents the social mask that everyone wears in public. From the Latin persona, human being, person, personage can be a part in a drama, an assumed character, or originally was conceived as a mask, or a false face.

Mask and persona point in the direction of social appearances and norms, and the imaginary ego, as a false master and cogito, and refer to saving and hiding the face from the gaze and scrutiny of the Other. It is precisely here where the two meanings of mask and semblance come to refer to the signifier. The subject uses social language or mythical narratives to conceal or reveal, in a distorted way, the unconscious signifying chain. In Poe's story this refers to how Lacan says that the effect or trajectory of the letter is being parodied by the false master or cogito making attempts to claim or affect its itinerary.

But can the "semblance" aspect of the signifier, the social mask, and the ego be bypassed? Can the signifier or desire function without a semblance in a direct and authentic fashion without distortion or displacement? This refers to the differences between psychoanalysis and existentialism or existential analysis since the existential notion of authenticity seems to presume a transparent or direct relationship between the subject and language. Given the metaphoric and metonymic structure of language, to express truth in language always requires a certain amount of fiction. In this sense the semblance of the signifier cannot be entirely bypassed. The semblance or mask or how the subject uses the signifier and social speech as a form of defense cannot be entirely avoided. Instead, the semblance has to be put to constructive use, from symptom to what Lacan comes to call the sinthome.

Appearance and persona also have semantic links in different languages. In English the word "a-pparent" as a homophone is related to being "a parent", and the word person as mask refers to each son (per-son). Between a parent and a son there is a relationship of kinship that in Spanish is written with the word "parentezco" that connotes a likeness or similarity of appearance (parecido) usually reflected in the semblant, or face. Between a parent and an offspring there is a likeness or kinship or relationship of identification that is usually reflected in the semblant.

The relationship of identification between parent and offspring is one between signifier and signified concatenated or linked by the law rather than by the satisfaction of needs. The child does not identify with the parent because the parent, like an animal parent, satisfies the child's needs, but because the parent represents the law that establishes the link between signifiers and the generations. When the signifier represents the subject, the subject is subjected and alienated under the signifier which is only a semblance of the subject's desire. The subject's unconscious desire appears concealed as implied for the signifier presented in the form of a social semblance.

By making a distinction between a letter in the Real and a symbolic signifier (12/5/71-p.VII 14), Lacan reflects on the possible existence of a discourse based on the letter and its relationship to the littoral (littorality and lituraterre). A littoral is the meeting place between two elements (water and land, jouissance and language) that mutually circumscribe each other. A letter represents the objet a that the Other has left behind or lost, and that re-appears in the figures of the subject's speech, in vibrant alliterations, erasures and obliterations of speech, and the portal through which jouissance both enters and escapes language. The expression "busy as a bee", for example, is an alliteration that adds elation, enthusiasm, desire, and enjoyment to a sentence. Every discourse is discursive, but a discourse can also be used in a non-discursive fashion through the Real aspect of the letter, the heart of the signifier, as a living and lively unit of speech (jouissance in words).

Syllepsis and catachresis are other examples of litterality, as a meeting place between the signifier and jouissance within language. In syllepsis, the expression "She lost it", for example, refers to a woman's or a man's temper, and whatever object "it" could indicate or be an index of. Black sun is the catachresis that bears the title of Kristeva's book on depression, and the experience of jouissance or suffering that a depressed person has to bear. Alternatively, and conversely, "luminous hole" could be used to describe the experience of mania or euphoria.

The question of the letter and the possibility of a discourse that would not be a semblance implies that the letter, perhaps, then, would not be a semblance or at least would be more Real than a signifier. The signifier represents an appearance and the letter something Real? This formulation or conclusion, however, runs the risk of replacing the duality between appearance and reality with a duality between the signifier and the letter. Nevertheless, such conclusion is already refuted by the Lacanian aphorism that truth or reality has the structure of fiction. There is a letter in the signifier, since words are made of letters, and letters are also an elementary unit of the signifier. The Real and the Symbolic, the letter and the signifier, are intersected in the Borromean knot.

However, at this point it is important to underscore a distinction between the true and truth, and between external reality and the Real. So-called true representations have the structure of fiction since representational truth takes place within a field of contested "truths". Reality for the symbolic semblant represents the true in the form of a fiction, in the sense of how Bentham and utilitarianism define fiction as an approximation or a probability that a representation could be true. The Real, instead, is the truth or the thing itself that the true is approximating, except that it lies outside and beyond the symbolic order. The Symbolic has the structure of fiction.

> There is confirmed the fact that the truth only progresses, only progresses from a structure of fiction.

Although Truth, as such, exists outside the signifier, such a truth does not have ontological existence outside the signifier or the Borromean knot. Truth is only true in emptiness. Otherwise, emptiness appears as a semblance. This is why Lacan says that truth only progresses from a structure of fiction. In fact, progress itself is a fiction for Lacan. What you gain on one side, you lose in the other. Revolutions are not necessarily progress or evolution; they could simply be disguised repetitions, or even forms of structural devolution or decay. A progress is achieved in one area that could cause other necessary areas of human experience to regress or collapse.

Letters are the point of contact between the signifier and the Real of jouissance within which the thing in itself is situated. The Real is a disruption for the stability of the signifier, or a form of senselessness in meaning, as well as an element of cohesion and consistency. Every letter can be erased or disrupted by the effect of a flux or wave of jouissance that it fails to represent. Letters as jouissance enter into language as a form of absence of representation contained within representation. On the other hand, such flux of jouissance outside representation animates the letter and brings fuel, cohesion, and linking to its function, as represented by how free association and interpretation work in the practice of analysis.

What is forgotten in representation is the aspect of truth in the Real, or of the subject's being and jouissance that fails to enter into or is subtracted from a true representation. In the spoken word, truth in the Real, has to be forgotten to be said, or said by not saying it, or by "naysaying" "it's not that" within the field of representation. As the ancient Chinese poet Tao Yuanming says: "beneath these things something real hides, but it dies on the tongue when I try to speak".

Finally, and as we said in the beginning of this section, the signifier as a semblance refers to the imaginary of saving face and finding protection from the gaze, and scrutiny of the Other with the use of language. The signifier as a semblance corresponds to what Lacan says about the effect or trajectory of the letter being parodied by the false master or cogito making attempts to claim or affect its itinerary.

> This "purloining of the letter" [vol de la lettre] will be said to be the parody of my discourse, whether one confines one's attention to the etymology of "parody," which indicates an accompaniment and implies the precedence of the trajectory that is parodied, or, in returning to the usual meaning of the term, one sees the shadow of the intellectual master dispelled in it in order to obtain the effect that I prefer to it.

The priority of the signifier, which is embodied as a trajectory or direction, as the choice of a particular signifying path that will reveal but defile neither the signifier nor the subject. The letter, with its displacement, its detour, traces out this path of the signifier, the symbolic movement. It is the symbolic movement of the letter more than instinctual impulses that drives the subject into actions. Dupin's "reminiscences" refer to Dupin's recollections of his history with the Minister and the Queen, while his "re-membering" refers to his rearranging of the signifying elements of the Purloined Letter to resolve the "police mystery story". Without the subject knowing about it, or in the shadow of the intellectual master, as Lacan says, the parody, in a story and in the subject's memory, becomes a secondary process, in order to resolve a police story and to make the parody lawful in conscious social life.

Remembering in the story is automatically defensive or more of a reminiscence than true remembering as discovered in analysis. Remembering is not only for purposes of resolving conflictual situations with others, but of signifying both desires, the Other's desires, and the defenses built against them. The Minister wanted to extort the Queen not so much for money, but to settle political differences and perhaps his jealousy as well. Dupin, for his part, wanted to receive a bounty from the Minister as well as seek revenge for past insults and injuries. But neither takes responsibility for their desire as an analysand would in their analysis. For this reason, we say that the story in its entirety remains within the grip of automaton. Only when the automaton of the letter is used to reveal something new about the subject's desire, while not compelling the subject to compulsive and pre-determined action, can one observe the workings of the undetermined and surprising Tyche as a principle of true chance and change.

Ultimately, the master of knowledge (Dupin and the Minister the poet), or connaissance as Lacan would call it, turns out to be only an effect of the symbolic order and the more he tends to rationalize his actions, the more his ego is shadowed by the signifiers. Both Minister D and Dupin fall into the trap of entering into the dark from the bright. Connaissance is ego knowledge and the brightness of discrimination, but the brightness does not allow us to see into the hidden structure of Beiing.

Lacan says, "Just so does the Purloined Letter, like an immense female body, sprawl across the space of the Minister's office when Dupin enters it". Entering the office as if into a woman's body refers to the Minister's jealousy, desire for the Queen, and the imaginary phallus (signifier of phallic privilege). Here the Purloined Letter, fully exposed there with its female disguise, turns to eat its own tail by Dupin's detection of Minister D's fantasy. And Dupin, with his excessive reasoning and narcissistic seeking of revenge, gives himself to the symbolic determination by enclosing the repetition loop. The repetition loop for Dupin is that the Minister also represents an Oedipal rival for Dupin, who is aligned with the mother Queen. Both of them are prey to automaton.

Poe's story represents something new in how he portrays the symbolic order and the discipline of the signifier functioning within a human story with all its cultural, symbolic, and sexual meanings. In reflecting upon the cultural fate of the letter and the signifier, Poe goes beyond automaton by outlining its very structure operation. Lacan's novelty lies in showing the structure of desire, fantasy, and censorship embedded within the signifying text. In addition, Lacan shows how the intellectual resolution of a mystery, or approaching the mystery from the bright side, only conceals the characters' true desires and motivation.

In our contribution, both Tyche and the experience of a personal analysis are required to reveal the curative aspects of the psychoanalytic understanding of a narrative, myth, or literary story. In Poe's story, the letter and detective story have a good social outcome thanks to Dupin's intellectual manipulations, but the truth of any of the character's desire remains undisclosed. When psychoanalysis is used to understand the story in terms of desire and social repression and power, and how these are intrinsic to the metaphoric and metonymic structure of language, this not only has the intellectual benefit of knowledge, but also refers to the therapeutic and emotional quality of insight and understanding as a form of knowing, savoir, or jouissance. However, the latter are more likely to be experienced and manifest in a personal analysis, rather than in the reading of a literary text, however enjoyable or tedious this may be.

If English literature was supposed to be the secular replacement for the educational and socializing aspect of Victorian religion, or for the "salvational" and moralizing quality of a religious text, an ingenious detective story can provide an interesting intellectual pastime, marred as it is with intrigues involving forbidden pleasures and corrupt forms of power, and this could in fact provide a release valve function for the repressions, desires, and conflicts, available and stimulated by the culture.

However, the experience of analysis goes beyond being a release valve function given that access to the lived experience of a subject's desire and jouissance leads to the possible emergence of something new within both psychical/subjective and objective linguistic structure. What the subject truly wants, or the subject's actual desire, is now reached through the inverted ladder of the law of symbolization that not only stops painful forms of jouissance but also becomes a pure form of desire representing the subject as a benevolent form of the Third jouissance.

References

Freud, S. (1909). Notes upon a Case of Obsessional Neurosis. *SE*, 10, 153–249.

Freud, S. (1920). Beyond the Pleasure Principle. New York: Norton, 1961

Freud, S. (1925). Negation. *SE*, 19, 235–239.

Heidegger, M. (1943). On the Essence of Truth. In *Basic Writings* (Revised and Expanded Edition). D.F. Krell (Trans.). London: Routledge, 1993.

Hofstadter, D. (1979). *Gödel, Escher, Bach: An Eternal Golden Braid*. New York: Basic Books, 1999.

Hume, D. (1748). Enquiry Concerning Human Understanding. In *Harvard Classics*, 37, Part 3. New York: Bartleby, 2001.

Hurst, A. (2008). Derrida Vis—vis Lacan: Interweaving Deconstruction and Psychoanalysis. New York: Fordham University Press.

Lacan, J. (2016). The Sinthome. London: Polity Press.

Lacan, J (1953–1954). Seminar I on the Technique of Psychoanalysis. London: Norton & Norton.

Lacan, J. (1971–1972). *...ou pire (Or Worse)*. Book XIX. Unpublished translation by C. Gallagher. www.lacaninireland.com.

Lacan, J. (1971)...on a discourse that would not be semblance. Translated by Cormac Gallagher from unedited French manuscripts.

Chapter 5

The Turn of the Screw and Lacan's Seminar XIV on the Logic of the Fantasy

Just like what was written for the first chapter, the purpose of this chapter is not to offer yet another additional interpretation of the text, nor shall we follow the same literary analytic method used by Lacan. We said that Lacan begins his text on "The Purloined Letter" by introducing relevant analytic concepts that will be employed for the study of a literary text, and then continues with a page-by-page analysis of the text interspersed with an elucidation of psychoanalytic ideas that could help carry the analysis of the text further. Our method will be different, and the purpose of this chapter is not simply to review and critique what other authors have said about the story and provide yet another interpretation, however accurate it may be.

For this chapter we do not have a Lacanian text on the "The Turn of the Screw" to analyze and comment upon. In addition, the topic of the fantasy is one without periodicity within Lacanian theory. Lacan's Seminar on the logic of the phantasy (XIV) is late enough to include most of what Lacan will say about the phantasm in his work. In this chapter, no distinction will be made between the middle period and the later period of Lacan's work.

This chapter will be divided into a plot summary, followed by a psychoanalytic analysis and a review of the psychoanalytic literature available on James' text. But the bulk of the chapter will be dedicated to using James' text for an in-depth analysis of Lacan's Seminar on the Logic of the Fantasy. This analysis of the Seminar will be focused more on the logical structure of the fantasy than on the mathematics of the golden number that Lacan also uses in Seminar XIV. The reason for this is that Moncayo has already written about Lacan's use of the golden and imaginary numbers in his prior two books.

Background and Plot Summary

There is no agreement on what exactly Henry James meant by "The Turn of the Screw". Some consider it a story of child abuse or neglect, of angelic and malevolent children, or a tale warning against overindulgence. Others have considered the story to be a straightforward ghost story.

Like Joyce, Yeats, Eliot, and others, James believed that the traditional rights of the creative imagination were infringed upon by the empirical spirit of scientific

DOI: 10.4324/9781003424574-5

culture. Oscar Wilde (1891) also wrote an essay "The Decay of Lying" where he laments the decay of the creative imagination. However, when psychoanalysis is included in the empirical spirit of contemporary scientific culture, then the creative imagination revealed in a literary work can also be used to reveal rather than conceal the structure of imaginary fantasies in human relations and experience. James believed in the power of nineteenth-century fiction to register and comment on the "the life of the times". James' imagination asserts itself primarily through a profound analytical sense of language and an exceptional dramatical power.

Since science rejects concerning itself with the subjective dimensions of human experience, such as sexual fantasy life, only literature can reveal the imaginary structure of human experience that otherwise remains inaccessible to the study methods of science or the social mores of society. In fact, many have charged James with sexual vulgarity in his writings. In addition, others consider it a study of evil and of the bottomless pit that accurses the human heart and mind. Literary art is being used to give a subtle account of human defilement. The notion of evil in the story includes death, the sexual abuse of children, the potential for madness in the human mind, and the belief in spirits and the afterlife. The diabolic value of the specters in "The Turn of the Screw" is almost invariably connected with their sexuality both in life and in death.

Henry James' story was dismissed by many as a detestable "Freudian affair", as if, if one rejected Freud, one could also outright dismiss the Turn of the Screw. The designation of the story as "Freudian" refers to how a story can arouse subjective responses in the reader. "The Turn of the Screw" was seen as a literary protest against the oppression and domination of modern life. What is damned about the story is the influence on the children exerted by Quint and Jessel. These descriptions are consistent with an interpretation of the story in which the governess would be driven to oppress the children because of her own unconscious conflicts. The governess's conflicts could be traced not only to Oedipal and psychical structure, but also to the social and economic inequities of Victorian Britain. For Edmund Wilson (1934) the ghosts in the story were not real ghosts but merely the governess's fantasies and hallucinations.

Similarly, Virginia Woolf believed the novel depicted the power of the human mind to reveal the ghosts haunting the mind and the structure of human desire. Others have argued (Reed, 1949) that the word psychical does not refer to unconscious fantasies but to the belief in the afterlife, ghosts, and their apparitions in the world of the living. These were things that Henry James' brother William studied while president of the Society for Psychical Research.

What all artists need, and what American artists and intellectuals only seem to be able to obtain by some conflict with the culture, is freedom from practical obligations and from the intellectual prejudice and social ties which could interfere with their creative vision. For the typical middle class American, intellectual interests are for the most part subordinated to moral, practical, and business interests. North American cultural surroundings have the effect of diluting the passion for intellectual purposes. As T. S. Eliot (1918) said regarding Henry James: there will always be a few intelligent people to understand any serious form of intellectual work, and to be understood by a few intelligent people is all the influence a person requires. In this chapter, we hope to explore in what sense the story is a serious intellectual creation from the perspective of psychoanalysis.

Written in 1898, Screw tells the story of a governess who takes a job with a man, who has been handed guardianship of his niece and nephew after they were orphaned in India. She is so overcome by his physical attractiveness that she feels compelled to take the job. The uncle strikes up a pretty sweet deal for her with one condition: that she must handle any issues that come up with the children and that he is not to be bothered under any circumstances. The governess heads off into the middle of nowhere to take care of Flora and Miles.

Upon arrival, the governess finds the house haunted by two ghosts who turn out to be Ms. Jessel, the children's last governess, and Peter Quint, a former servant of the uncle. In life they were a couple and cared for Miles and Flora. Both died under mysterious circumstances. Ms. Jessel's cause of death is unknown, and Quint was found dead on the side of the road from a blow to the head, perhaps from slipping on the ice. Convinced that the ghosts are a threat to the children, the governess sends Flora away with Mrs. Grose when she comes down with a fever, leaving her and Miles alone in the house.

When Peter Quint reappears, the governess immediately starts screaming for him to leave Miles alone, that the children are hers and that he must stop tormenting them. Miles, seemingly unaware of Quint's presence, asks Quint and then responds, Oh Quint, you devil! As he rushes to the window to confront him, the governess pulls him back, holding him and telling him everything will be alright. As Quint falls away from view, the governess realizes that the child she's holding in her arms is dead.

Quint is really a threat: he lures Miles to the window in order to kill him and to take him back into the spirit realm, or perhaps he kills Miles because he can't have him.

Neither Mrs. Grose, nor Miles, nor Flora ever admits to seeing Peter Quint or Ms. Jessel. The governess is really the only person who claims to see them and reacts to their presence in the house. This raises the question whether the entire play is a product of her fantasies with the ghosts representing her fantasized sexuality both with her employer and with the children who are used to enhance her potential sexual life with her employer.

From the beginning, the governess claims ownership of the children, calling them my children, or my Miles, etc. She claims she's dazzled by their loveliness and makes a commitment that she will charm their uncle into coming back through her dedication. The children will be her objet a, or what completes her through solving the problem with the children for the uncle, and she hopes this will endear her to him. She hints that if she can control the children for long enough, perhaps she can insinuate herself into the family. We know very little of the governess's background aside from the fact that she's desperate for work and willing to do anything to impress the uncle. She falls in love with Miles and Flora so quickly that it seems as if she's replacing a missing child with them. Through the children she seeks to become an object of desire for the uncle.

Although this is a Lacanian reading of the story, this was already anticipated by Wilson (1934) in his study on Henry James.

> The writer posits that "the ghosts are hallucinations of the governess" (p. 171), and that her insistence on her own delusions not only causes the two kids to dislike her but it also leads Miles to be killed by her; "[s]he has literally frightened him to death" (p. 172). Wilson writes that the governess has a disturbed personality. It is stated that she cannot acknowledge "her sexual impulses" (p. 172); this shows that The Turn of the Screw is not a ghost story but "a study in morbid psychology" (p. 172). Wilson argues that only through this way of reading we can observe a consistency among Henry James's literary works around his acquainted theme of "frustrated Anglo-Saxon spinster" (p. 173).
> (https://taqienglish.blogspot.com/2017/12/the-ambiguity-of-henry-james.html)

Another popular interpretation is that Quint was perhaps sexually abusive to Miles in life and has come back from the dead to claim him once again. Benjamin Britten's operetta adaptation of the same name certainly suggests this reading.

James' ghost story emphasizes the class conflicts within society. Quint and Jessel's roles as servants and unexplained deaths are linked to their aggressive spirits desperate maneuver to take hold of the children. They are pitted against the governess's same desperation to find her desire and happiness as Miles and Flora's caregiver. Miles and Flora are victims of imperialism, their parents having died in India, without a family member to care for them. The governess, then, in destroying what she hoped to live for, is left alone. Without the children she has no livelihood. And thus continues the turn of the screw or the tragedy of the working class and the tragedy of human sexuality.

At the very beginning of the story, it says, "A ghost story with one child in it is frightening enough. But two children who see ghosts – isn't that quite strange? Doesn't that give the story another turn of the screw?" A ghost story with a child in it is frightening and becomes even more frightening with two kids in it. Why does the appearance of a kid or kids make the story more horrible? Is it because it accords with the concept of the uncanny, causing the effect of the familiar turning into the unfamiliar, or vice versa? Anyway, here the word "turning" is very important. It can mean the increase of tensions; at the same time, it also means a subtle transformation in psychical reality.

Analysis

The novel addresses the questions of the human sexual drive and childhood sexuality, and how they conflict with cultural rules. One character in the play (Quint) is conceived as a libertine from a lower class that incites and perverts the childhood sexuality in the children known as Miles and Flora. The working-class governess is in love with her upper-class master/employer who could not be bothered with her or his niece and nephew. The uncle is not a true uncle, who can pass for and function as a parent. The parent employer in this case could not care less, mirroring conditions that critics have said about capitalist social relations.

Apparently, the governess has never had children and sees the children as her extensions that complete her in her wishes to be desired by an employer who does not want to parent the children. The uncle is detached and uninterested in the children's problems who lost their parents and are orphans. The libertine/pervert character was a younger man before he died who had also seduced the previous governess who also died and was in love with him despite being from an upper class. Like the first governess went down in class in her object choice, perhaps because the uncle, whom she was also interested in, also rejected her. The second governess set her sights in choosing a lover from a higher class than hers.

The book is also an English ghost story like many others. Ghosts here are featured as haunting the children due to how their sexual and romantic excesses and choices in life led to their death, and how these may have included caretakers sexually abusing children who willingly participated in it. Quint and Ms. Jessell's fantasy life led to their deaths, making obvious the links between forbidden sex and death. Both sexual life and death are the source of many imaginative fantasies.

It is said that ghosts are spirits who cannot proceed to the spirit world due to unfinished and unresolved sexual and aggressive transgressions in this world while they were alive. Despite the punishment of death, Quint still insists on having an inappropriate relationship with a child. Ghosts as living dead people, and fantasies or fantasy life, have in common that they drive human beings to pursue their wishes despite the law, and despite death.

The story also shows how the children function as fantasy and wish fulfillment for the governess who seeks to become more attractive to the uncle through the children. In a way she has the children with her lover before her lover wishes to have sex with her and without knowing whether he will ever be interested in her, which seems unlikely.

The story also shows the contradictory ways of viewing childhood in Western culture. Children are both angelic and pure, and at the same time capable of what Freud called childhood sexuality consisting mostly of fantasies and sexual satisfaction unrelated to procreation, since this is something that happens before puberty and biological maturation. Freud referred to this as the polymorphous perversion of childhood where, like in sexual aberrations, sexuality is unlinked to marriage and reproduction. However, in childhood sexuality under normal circumstances there is no knowledge or disavowal of the law and therefore this kind of sexuality can be seen as innocent despite its perverse overtones. Perhaps this is similar to how animals publicly engage in sexual intercourse as something completely natural without apparent conflict with social or moral values. In fact, perverts often appeal to this fact to lower the resistances of their victims.

Beautiful children can be both angelic and naughty or malevolent at the same time. The book makes clear that malevolence is tied to their beauty and their bodies, and not only due to the sexual abuse of others. At the same time the book seems to attribute uncivilized sexuality to the lower classes while not sparing the upper classes either who are neglectful, not only with the workers, but also with their children.

To understand the connections and differences between fantasy and phantasm or ghost, and between childhood sexuality and the perversion of children, we need to begin with an introduction to psychoanalytic theory that has had many things to say about these matters. Psychoanalytic theory will be introduced from the specific perspective of unconscious fantasy, which, in our opinion, is the most relevant psychoanalytic concept to understand the coherence and consistency of James' story.

Lacan's Seminar XIV on The Logic of the Phantasy or Phantasm.

The notion of the phantasm (another term for ghost) in Lacan dates back to Freud's (1915, 1916–1917; Laplanche and Pontalis, 1973) "protofantasies" or "primal fantasies", which included the question of the origins: the origins of sexuality or the seduction fantasy; the question of castration, or the origin of sexual differences; and the primal scene, or the origin of human life. According to Freud (1915, 1916–1917), these universal structures exist in a fantasy dimension and are irreducible to personal individual experience (a point that Jung borrowed). This means that people experience fantasies but the experience is not unique to them.

According to Lacan, unconscious fantasy both sustains desire and defends against prohibition or what is technically known in psychoanalysis as symbolic castration. "What is prohibited is always present in the actual formation of the wish" (Laplanche and Pontalis, 1973). The crossing of the phantasm or fantasy involves elaborating on these two aspects of the fantasy: how the fantasy sustains desire and at the same time defends against symbolic castration.

We will pause and explain what is meant by castration within Lacanian theory in this day and age. Castration, for Freud, referred to a fantasized mutilation or dismemberment of the penis that established the psychical differences between the sexes. According to Freud, both sexes reject femininity due to the perceived fantasized castration of the mother: the mother does not have a penis because she lost it. Lacan gives more weight to the castration complex at the same time that he gives it a more structural, mathematical, and symbolic interpretation. In addition, the object of the symbolic lack, resulting from the operation of symbolic castration, is the imaginary phallus, and not the penis.

The allegedly anatomical absence of the penis in the mother refers to the symbolic condition whereby the child represented an imaginary phallic and narcissistic object for the mother. The father intervenes and breaks the fantasized fusion and thus symbolically "castrates" both mother and child. The child will no longer be an imaginary phallus for the mother, and the child becomes a subject in his/her own right. From then on, the demand for the phallus will be addressed to the father, and the omnipotence of the mother is transferred to the father.

However, at first, Lacan located the lack in the Other in the mother and considered that the father actually possessed the imaginary phallic attribution.

For example, in Lacan's interpretation of Desire in Hamlet, Hamlet's father in Shakespeare's prose is presented as having the imaginary phallus in Hamlet's speech.

> See what a grace was seated on this brow,
> Hyperion's curls, the front of Jove himself,
> An eye like Mars' to threaten and command,
> A station like the herald Mercury
> New-lighted on a heaven-kissing hill,
> A combination and a form indeed
> Where every god did seem to set his seal
> To give the world assurance of a man.
> This was your husband.

With his later studies on the Name of the Father and the symbolic phallus/function, Lacan comes to understand that the lack in the Other also applies to the father, however necessary the imaginary phallic attribution may be at a certain moment of the child's development. But Lacan, as far as we can tell, never went back to revise his theory of Oedipal phases/moments. Thus, Moncayo (2008) has argued for a fourth moment/phase of Oedipus where the omnipotence of the father is also necessarily lost at some point.

Castration for Lacan ultimately is negotiated in relationship to the lack in the (f)Other and the realization that the phallus (and the Other) does not exist and was never there more than as a function, and this leads to the possibility of going beyond the bedrock of castration. This was Lacan's work of the early seventies, particularly in … ou pire (*Or Worse...*, Seminar XIX, 1971–1972a) and The Knowledge of the Psychoanalyst (*Seminar XIXa*, 1971–1972b).

For Lacan, the symptom is necessary to access unconscious fantasies. As we will explain below, fantasy is an image set in a repressed and unconscious signifying structure. Fantasies may be repressed, acted out, or perceived as elements of the external world. In addition, fantasies veil the lack or the desire of and in the Other (not the desire for the Other). Since the desire of the Other or what the other wants from the subject is an enigma, the subject produces the fantasy as a fantasized answer of the subject to the question, "What does the Other want from me?" A fantasy represents a veil upon the lack in the form of an answer that comes back to the subject in inverted form (back from the Other although it is the subject's own answer). The Other or Society wants to take a pound of flesh from the subject (an imaginary castration fantasy based on symbolic castration). Projection is different, because projection is the exposition of the lack in the Other, rather than the subject.

For example, in the story we find the following passage:

> "Certainly. I stay on as your friend and from the tremendous interest I take in you till something can be done for you that may be more worth your while. That needn't surprise you." My voice trembled so that I felt it impossible to suppress

> the shake. "Don't you remember how I told you, when I came and sat on your bed the night of the storm, that there was nothing in the world I wouldn't do for you?"
>
> (James, H. (1898) The Turning of the Screw. Public Domain. p.106)

Here we find the enigma of desire. What do the adult and the child want from each other that might be "worth their while". The surprising desire, if forbidden, should not surprise the subject in an attempt to make such desires acceptable. What the adult wants to do for the child does not seem to have any limits. Regarding Quint's desire, the governess says, "I've never seen one like him. He did what he wished". "With her?" "With them all". "Too free with my boy?" "Too free with everyone!" This represents the fantasy of the imaginary unbarred master "who dares all things" to the extent that no human beings can actually be. In reference to this Lacan says, "This allows us to see the imaginary import of the personage" (Ecrits, p. 24).

Although fantasies have common elements, they are always singular formations of the subject. Fantasies also often come in contradictory pairs that in the case of hysteria are exemplified by bisexuality and the question of hysteria, according to Lacan: "Am I a man or a woman, am I both a man and a woman, or neither (three possible rational/logical levels)". In addition, the fantasy, or phantasm, as Lacan called it, is staged in the choice of one or two simultaneous and contradictory partners of the different or same sex. For Lacan hysteria since Freud has always been two.

What is the logic of phantasy, and how is fantasy an important yet variable and surprising reference point in the psyche? This chapter is an elucidation, commentary, and elaboration of Lacan's Seminar XIV (66–67) on The Logic of the Phantasm. Gallagher's version of the seminar is the only unedited translation from original recordings of Lacan's oral teaching of the Seminar, and available for free in the "Lacan in Ireland" website. In this chapter, we will focus on key concepts that Lacan discusses in this Seminar.

We will begin from the writing of the fantasy, namely, from the formula: S barred diamond small a ($ ◇a). The S barred ($) represents that the subject is barred from the object of desire and feels barred by the presence of the object, and by the repressive unconscious operation. The inhibition and anxiety (effects of the bar or of the subject being barred) experienced in the presence of the object of desire refers back to the objet a cause of desire that has been lost due to the bar of the Law. In addition, the subject also feels barred by the unconscious repressive operation because it lies outside the sphere of the ego's conscious control.

The formula for the fantasy establishes a connection between the subject and something else, which is called small a. The relation between desire and the object of desire is a logical relation properly speaking. The diamond, pointer, or rhomboid ◇ represents the logical relations among the terms. If we draw a horizontal line across the symbol, then we discover the functions of separation in the lower half (V) of the symbol (◇), and conjunction or fusion (A) in the upper half. If we draw a vertical line across the diamond, then we find the arithmetical and logical functions of less than (<) and more than (>).

So, with the diamond there are four vectors: fusion, separation, more, and less. The first two refer to the state of the connection between the subject and the objet a, the latter two refer to the extent or magnitude of this connection. The four vectors constitute four possible imaginary sets of fantasy (separation and more, separation and less, fusion and more, fusion and less). In fact, these sets may represent the differences between subjects in how they experience separation and fusion within a relationship. Desire in the fantasy also finds its reference point in the visual imaginary insofar as the beloved other of a relationship is seen through the logical eyes of the fantasy.

The term fantasy suggests a relation to fantasia, to the imagination. But the fact remains that fantasy and logic are not so fundamentally, so radically opposed to one another as one might first think. Moreover, the imaginary feature of what is called the objet a will appear as a logical value much less related, at first sight, to the domain of what is properly speaking the Imaginary. The Imaginary, rather, is attached to it, surrounds it, accumulates in it. Logic is symbolic not imaginary, yet the imaginary surrounds and envelops logic.

Lacan argues the thesis that the fantasy is structured like a language in a narrower sense than the rest of the unconscious. The fantasy is a sentence with a grammatical structure, and thus capable of articulating the logic of the fantasy. Lacan poses it as a form of predicate logic where a sentence expresses a proposition that must be true or false.

In mathematical logic, a sentence (or closed formula) of a predicate logic is a Boolean-valued well-formed formula with no free variables. A sentence can be viewed as expressing a proposition, something that must be true or false. For this reason, Lacan used the specific form of predicate logic to understand the logical structure of the fantasy that the subject experiences as a fixed or frozen reality. Fantasy is only concerned with the values true or false.

Freud writes the fantasy "a child is being beaten" as it is written in German – not "one beats a child", for example. "A child is being beaten" appears as a grammatically structured sentence. In the structure of a neurosis, this fantasy is not linked specifically to the subject or the other. It is unclear who is being beaten or who is doing the beating. Typically, it is a brother or a sister who is getting beaten. Eventually it becomes clear that it is the father who is doing the beating. "My father is beating the child whom I hate, and this means that he loves only me". Secondarily, "My father is beating me not my brother". So, it seems that in Freud's sentence, the subject and the object can be filled with variables. Is this contradictory with Lacan's use of predicate logic for the formula, or are they stating different aspects of the fantasy? I think, Freud stresses the replacement of subjects and the others in the sentence. But the truth value, as Lacan states, is always true or false.

The formula can also be applied to the case of anorexia. As one of our colleagues has observed in the therapeutic practice with anorexia, the anorexic loves to watch others eat more than they need, especially her parents, although she herself seldom eats. "My father/mother is eating the food I hate. I am being hated by my parents".

The form of the fantasy is sadistic; its satisfaction is masochistic. To derive satisfaction from watching others eat beyond what is healthy or satisfying is sadistic, while feeling guilty about eating or suffering as a result of it is masochistic. Guilt transforms sadism into masochism. The guilt refers not only to the act of masturbation linked to the fantasy but to the fantasy itself. It is unclear if the pleasure experienced in the beating is sadistic or masochistic. The fantasy is then transformed into "I am beaten by my father". The patient acknowledges that they are probably looking on. Girls observe their brothers being beaten, toward whom they experience sibling rivalry. Usually, it is boys that are beaten in the fantasies of girls as well. Subjects who have this fantasy preserve a dislike for father figures and are easily offended by them.

A fantasy of this kind is a primary trait of perversion. In the case of the wolfman Freud is referring to a perverse trait within a neurotic structure. A person with a perverse structure disavows the law, but more significantly and specifically, disavows the differences between the sexes. The prime example that Freud uses is fetishism found mostly in men for whom the interest in a woman is reduced to a shoe that proves that she has the phallus and therefore the difference between the sexes as such is disavowed. In perversion the fantasy is acted out rather than repressed.

The fantasy is acted out with demands for some fairly bizarre sexual practices. Joyce had the perverse trait of liking to watch his wife defecate and watch the feces come out of her anus. He had a psychotic structure according to Lacan, but this was a perverse trait. When it becomes a trait in childhood, a perverse trait like this does not last a lifetime. It will be transformed by repression, reaction formation, or sublimation. If these defenses do not take place, the perversion lasts to maturity. The disgust or pleasure in feces and defecation differentiates a neurotic from a perverse trait.

In the case "a child is being beaten" as it is written in German Freud notes that it often appeared in the cases of hysteria and obsessional neurosis that he treated. The fantasy has elements of pleasure attached to it and involves a masturbatory satisfaction. These fantasies are entertained in early childhood before school age. The children are being beaten for being naughty and for their bad conduct. The punishment should not do any serious injury. Subjects who had this fantasy were never actually beaten in their childhoods. Fantasy is a kind of dramatization of his/her life in the child's mind. What is its structural function? The function is the formation of material implication. In reality there is a loose connection between the premise and the conclusion, but the fantasy conditions the subject to draw from any premise the same conclusion. In this way, fantasy becomes a reality for the subject, and a source of disappointment for the subject because the fantasy they believe in never becomes true.

The characteristic of the false is that one deduces from it in the same step, on the same footing, the false and the true. This is why the camouflage or deception aspect of the fantasy has a logical structure. The false does not exclude the true. The fantasy, although false, includes the truth of the symptom, of psychical structure, and the signifying chain. There is no obstacle to a premise being false, provided its conclusion is true, for it to be classified with the index of truth. What in logic is called material implication requires only one thing: that the conclusion should be true.

That P implies Q can also be said by saying that not –P is divergent from Q, which is the same as saying that P is convergent with Q. P and Q are either divergent or convergent, so that if –P or not P is divergent from Q, then this means that P is convergent with Q. That ghosts imply sexuality is expressed in the sentences in such a way that removing sexuality from the equation would diverge from the topic of understanding the nature of ghosts. Sentences in the story where sexuality is discussed function as theorems for the theory that explains the narrative or the set of sentences from the point of view of the axioms. The sexual sentences in the story don't have to be true to function as theorems for the conclusion that the ghost story is linked to sexuality and childhood sexuality.

This definition of material implication does not imply that material implication only works if A strictly implies B only if it is impossible for both A and ~B to be true (strict formal implication). Psychoanalysis is more consistent with intuitionistic logic. In intuitionist logic, the implication $A \supset B$ is true if there exists a proof that, if conjoined to a proof of A, would produce a proof of B. Is there a proof of the subject that in the formula for the fantasy would be conjoined and produce a proof of the objet a? The subject is barred or divided by the prohibition of incest. The subject is the logical consequence of the bar that results in a symbolic exchange of objects and/or signifiers.

Fantasy exists upon at least two planes. One is the fundamental fantasies that support the subject. The prohibition of incest belongs to the primal fantasy. The primal fantasy is consistent with intuitionistic logic. There is another fantasy that is the result of the subject of desire or divided subject. Since the object of desire is lost, it has to be constructed upon the level of the subject. This is the fantasy sustaining the desire of the subject. But the second fantasy is more Cantorian than Brouwerian, because the second fantasy is the result of the logical sequence or the logical movement of the signifiers.

The proof of the existence of the prohibition of incest, and the proof of the existence of a divided subject (between prohibition and the object cause of desire), produces the proof that the object of desire in the fantasy, as a variable, is a lost or forbidden object of desire (objet a) that as a variable has been substituted for a new object in the fantasy. In addition, in the fantasy, the subject and the object conjunct, meaning that the subject implies the object, and the object implies the subject. However, this is not always true. Sometimes the subject and the object separate, and when they are disjunct and different, then one or the other may become more or less important to each other.

The logical links between a ghost story, sexuality, and childhood sexuality show how, in contrast to philosophy and science, psychoanalysis deals with ghosts, albeit also in a scientific manner proper to the subject of study. Specters that inhabit psychical reality constitute the object or, more precisely, the subject of psychoanalysis. However, it is not only psychoanalysis that is inhabited by ghosts as demonstrated by the James novel that serves as an example of literary modernism.

Another example of a fantasy/dream is found in Freud's the case of the wolfman.

> I dreamt that it was night and that I was lying in bed. Suddenly, the window opened of its own accord, and I was terrified to see that some white wolves were sitting on a big walnut tree in front of the window. There were six or seven of them. The wolves were quite white and had big tails and had their ears pricked like dogs when they pay attention to something. In great terror, evidently of being eaten up by the wolves, I screamed, and woke up.

The white wolves remind him of sheep who are eaten by wolves. His father would take him to see sheep, and sometimes he would playfully threaten to "gobble him up". His sister, who was his father's favorite, used to scare him showing him pictures of wolves. When it became obvious that she was her father's favorite, he was devastated. "Many years later she killed herself, and I hardly felt a trace of grief". The tree also referred to a story he heard of someone being attacked by wolves.

In his "naughty period", Pankejeff's masochism was at the forefront of his relation to his father. This was in focus on the night of the dream. The terms sadism and masochism came from the language of the sexual aberrations classified by sexologist Kraft Ebbing at the turn of the twentieth century. S&M refers to contractual sexual sadomasochistic practices, but Freud made sadism and masochism normal vicissitudes of the drive, alongside seeing and being seen (voyeurism and exhibitionism).

It is commonly held that sadism is prior to masochism, and that masochism is sadism turned around upon the subject's own self. In fact, sadism in this context has the sense of an aggression against the other person in which the other's suffering is not a relevant factor. Psychoanalysis would appear to show that the infliction of pain plays no part among the original aims and objects of the aggressive drive. The father's actions, for example, are not relevant to the son's decision of disavowing or not identifying himself with father. It is rather the son's fantasy about identification that makes the son disavow his father. Symbolic identification implies castration and for this reason it is disavowed. Here lies the logic of material implication. Because symbolic castration is experience as something false in the imaginary, identification is rejected.

> "Masochism corresponds to a turning round against the subject's own self and at the same time to a reversal of activity into passivity. Only with the masochistic period does the aggressive drive take on a sexual meaning, and only then does the infliction of suffering become intrinsic to this activity" (Laplanche and Pontalis, 1988, p. 402). Freud also wrote: "...Sensations of pain, like other unpleasurable sensations, trench upon sexual excitation and produce a pleasurable

> condition, for the sake of which the subject will even willingly experience the unpleasure of pain".
>
> (Freud, 1915, p. 128)

> Freud points out two stages in this process of turning round upon the self: in the first, the subject inflicts suffering on himself – an attitude particularly evident in obsessional neurosis; in the second, characteristic of masochism proper, the subject has pain inflicted upon himself by another person. Thus, before passing into the "passive" voice the verb "to inflict suffering" goes into the reflexive, "middle" voice: a child is being beaten, pain is being inflicted. Finally, sadism, in the sexual sense of the term, is achieved by virtue of another turning round of the masochistic position. In sadism, "while these pains are being inflicted on other people, they are enjoyed masochistically by the subject through the identification of the subject with the suffering object".
>
> (Laplanche and Pontalis, 1988, p. 402)

We said that in his "naughty period", Pankejeff's masochism was at the forefront of his relation to his father. This was in focus on the night of the dream. Pankejeff goes to sleep thinking of the Xmas presents on the tree. His dominant masochistic impulses find expression in the wish: the theme of "receiving" something from his father gets a passive, masochistic connotation.

All of a sudden, the two preoccupations converge: the primal scene of a child being beaten, or a child being bitten (homophony) by the signifier wolf, becomes sexualized, and a passive sexual feminine position in relation to his father is given terrifying new connotations.

In another similar example, an analysand reported that his mother told him that her younger brother was preferred over her by her parents for being a boy. On the one hand, she had to support her younger brother and, on the other hand, she hated her brother for being preferred and privileged over her. His mother used to enjoy when her brother got a beating for being spoiled and naughty. In addition, she enjoyed when her brother once got bitten by a snake because she felt it was justified due to his naughtiness. We find here the same homophony between being beaten and being bitten by a snake. Analysand reports that uncle always remained a boy and never grew up to be a man. The analysand's mother enjoyed seeing her brother being beaten and bitten by a phallic signifier rather than thinking of him as occupying an imaginary phallic privilege over her because he was a boy. In the beatings and the snake's bite, the brother suffers imaginary castration in the same way that she suffered imaginary castration by being treated as less than boys and her brother.

If Pankejeff's masochism implied a wish to be beaten by his father, the discovery of sexual difference turned this into a gendered position: the idea of being his father's woman. To be his father's woman would involve a terrifying loss. In Freud's account, Pankejeff woke up in a state of intense castration anxiety, which for the next six months was expressed in an oral register: as a terror of being eaten by a wolf.

With respect to the functioning of the signifier as a letter, Lacan gives the example of the figure of the Roman number five (V), as a signifier of desire, in so far as Roman number V, as a typographical element, could represent the outspread legs of a woman as a metaphor for the vagina or femininity, or the beating of the wings of a butterfly. The latter, in turn, can also be used to represent feminine jouissance more than femininity.

The way in which fantasy life and the truths of desire reveal a logical structure within the analytic process shows how the relation between the signifier and truth is by no means direct, transparent, or self-evident. We cannot transparently say the truth about the true! The T about the T, or the true about truth. The signifier cannot signify itself except precisely when it is not itself that it signifies, namely, when it uses metaphor. Truth discloses itself in constant substitutions. In the fantasy formula, the object of desire presents itself as a variable. And there is nothing to prevent the metaphor which substitutes a different signifier for the true of the Truth, from making the truth re-emerge at this moment, with the ordinary effect of metaphor, namely, the creation of a false signified. The rosy fingers of dawn to represent the sun, for example.

Predicate logic introduced by Aristotle points to the field that designates what lies inside and outside a given predicate. The inside and outside of a predicate mark a topological edge. Lacan does not believe to be saying the true about Truth, but, rather, that he is saying the true about what Freud said. Truth here not as a positive proposition, nor its negation (It is not true), but rather truth in the form of a double negation: "not without" truth. Fiction is not without truth, although it is not directly related to or descriptive of truth.

A child is being beaten is not true but is not without truth. Truth does not refer to the narrative of the story but to the way the unconscious signifier and its logic thinks for the subject (I am where it is not me who is doing the thinking: the Ucs. subject is thinking at a place where the ego is not, and the conscious ego is not thinking but simply being a witness to the workings of the signifying structure). There is no comprehension in the ego but what occurs instead is simply an extension of the work of the signifier into the larger mental and logical structure.

Another main feature of Freud's fantasy sentence is its present continuous tense: a child is being beaten. The present continuous tense represents the structure of logical and metonymic displacement. To be here now in the fantasy simply means to act on the basis of like and dislike, preference, or changing displaced feelings. One does not act on the basis of principle that may require a temporary postponement of satisfaction, but instead the subject and the signifier are like a raft drifting according to the tides and moods of the ocean. Here oceanic feeling means impulse or instinctual soup, rather than the sublated feelings associated with more convenient forms of jouissance.

Now is logical or symbolic structure the same as what Lacan calls a Universe of discourse? Are discourse, speech, and writing the same thing? A discourse can be written or spoken but in either case it is an authoritative statement, or a personal speech act, or enunciation. As a speech act, discourse also articulates and manifests a symbolic structure, while writing is related to the written language in a text. A discourse is a synchronic temporal structure, while writing, with its "ing" form, seems to capture the diachronic temporal element of language.

Discourse in psychoanalysis not only refers to a theory about psychical or linguistic structure. Discourse is also a speech act, or an enunciation in the here and now of an analytical session that reveals the structure of desire. Writing instead is an act that reflects the anterior future (of the potential reader) and the posterior past when the past will be read in the anterior future. The temporality of writing and speech differ.

Reading as speech gives new meaning and life to a text by transforming the moment of writing, which is also a speech act for the author, into the speech act of a reading subject. The temporality of speech and desire is transferred from the writer to the reader via the mediation represented by the perennial and atemporal appearance of a text. True, a text was written at a specific point in time, but then becomes eternal literature for the ages, with eternity here being defined as a period of time that lasts for a long time, but not forever.

In psychoanalysis, the temporality of speech is in the here and now, and it is closely intersubjective. The present temporality of writing is the posterior past and anterior future. At the time of writing, the author is in the presence of the authors that came before them, and in the presence of their future audience (anterior future), but not in the presence of another subject. Is any subject ever in the presence of another subject? In other words, is the other always an imaginary objet a for the subject? Not exactly, since the interaction with the social other is regulated by the structure of speech and language (the Other, or what in this case can be considered a symbolic form of intersubjectivity since subjects and not only signifiers are involved).

In this sense, an author's objet a, or an object's cause of desire, is metonymically represented by the characters in the story, just like in a dream the characters represent the ego of the dreamer. In a dream the objects of the subject that appear in the fantasy are represented by other subjects. But the other is not present when a subject is writing or dreaming. This differs from speech that usually has an interlocutor in the present moment.

Seen from these two temporalities, the analyst working in a session performs a different function than an ordinary interlocutor. When an analysand comes to see the analyst, at first they may refuse to speak in the presence of the analyst, or when they begin speaking they may not speak about themselves, and when they begin speaking about themselves they may not address the analyst. When they finally speak to the analyst about themselves, a logical termination may become possible. Thus, to reach a satisfactory conclusion, psychoanalysis requires what Lacan calls the traversal of the fantasy. The traversal of the fantasy refers to realizing its logical structure, accepting how it supports desire while not being fooled by it either, since the fantasy is also a defense formation against symbolic castration. This work is done in the intimacy of speech addressed to another, but, more importantly, to the Other of the Unconscious structure.

However, analysis is not mutual understanding, and there is always a dissymmetry in the temporality between analyst and analysand. The time of the analysand is that of the moment of speech where the signified in speech reveals the desire of the subject. While for the analyst, time is both of speech and of writing. Other than the analyst's interpretative and professional speech that reveals the subject's desire (not the analyst's desire), the temporality of the analyst speech is more like writing. More like writing, because the analyst does not seek a close intersubjective connection with the analysand based on the analyst's objects of desire. The analyst instead speaks out of a gap where both the posterior past and anterior future tenses reside and function. The gap or emptiness is where the present moment represents emptiness as well as the past and future.

Lacan says that it is no longer tenable to consider that there is a Universe of discourse, for there is something lacking in the signifying chain. This flaw in the Universe of discourse, or the lack in the symbolic order, is manifested at certain points of paradox that reveal an incomplete yet consistent system. The Symbolic refers to the consistent yet incomplete laws of language, society, myth, culture, and symbolic thought. The Imaginary refers to visual perception, fantasy life, and the ego of narcissism. The Real has two forms and periods in Lacan. For the early Lacan the Real was threatening to the symbolic order in the form of something traumatic and hazardous that disrupts and tears symbolic links. The second form of the Real, presented in Seminar XXIII, is a hole that organizes, structures, and generates accord and coherence within the Borromean knot. If you untie one of the rings the entire knot becomes untied. Lacan says that in analysis the knot needs to be untied and then retied into a new knot.

In Seminar RSI Lacan says three things about consistency: that there is consistency in each register, in the knot itself, and that consistency is the main characteristic of the Imaginary. The Real instead is characterized by "ex-istence", while the Symbolic makes a hole.

The Imaginary wants to create a consistent and complete world in two respects. With respect to the fantasy, consistency points to a fantasized situation being organized within the grammatical structure of a sentence. In visual perception, complete refers to the visual field being a saturated whole. In formalism in mathematics, Hilbert thought that arithmetic could be shown to be both complete and consistent. This was until Gödel showed that arithmetic is consistent because it is incomplete, and that complete systems are inconsistent.

The Symbolic is such a consistent and incomplete system. The Symbolic speaks the language of the underlying relations that determine perception and the conditions of intelligibility. In the Symbolic there are three kinds of consistencies. First, there is the consistency created by covering the hole or paradox inside the symbolic system itself. Second is the consistency of automaton generating predictable repetitions. Third is the consistency provided by material implication. The latter in logic implies that no matter how many fictions or fantasies the subject may have, this does not prevent them from being truths of desire. The truths of desire are not irrational because they have logical structure despite not having correspondence with reality.

The Borromean knot as a figure for mental structure is "holy" (has the nature of a hole) insofar as emptiness articulates its consistency. In this respect, the consistency of the Imaginary is false since the homogeneity and saturation of the visual field hides the signifiers and logarithms that give the images their consistency and functionality within language. What makes a system consistent is that some truths in it cannot be proven within the PM arithmetical system.

However, we cannot prove that the consistency of the Imaginary is false. The Imaginary is complete and yet inconsistent. On the surface, the Imaginary appears true and complete, but with Gödel we now know that if a system or register appears complete, then it must be inconsistent. Complete systems have the limitation that they cannot prove their own consistency. Only systems that cannot prove their own consistency are consistent. Consistent systems will always contain truths that cannot be proven within the system due to key elements being missing from the structure.

Arithmetic or the PM system is consistent because it is incomplete like the symbolic order. Some truths of arithmetic cannot be proven such as why imaginary or unreal numbers can provide real and precise solutions despite not existing. The consistency of the Imaginary requires outer proofs whether from the Symbolic or from the Real. The Real is consistent, while "ex-sisting", because it is a vacuum plenum without differentiations. In this sense, the vacuum plenum is like a sub-quantum vacuum state that provides a constancy and consistency for the universe.

The fantasy is the proof for the Imaginary. According to material implication, a fantasy does not have to be true in order to be true. The fantasy as a premise can be false, yet it leads to true conclusions regarding mental structure. The Borromean knot of four demonstrates the consistency of the Real as a form of Real concord or accord between the registers. The proof of the Symbolic lies in textual rigor and the logical articulation of signifiers. However, this articulation or tight link between signifiers is predicated on the fact that the elemental unit of the signifier is empty or cannot signify itself by itself. The emptiness of the signifier is the area of intersection between the Real and the Symbolic.

Returning to the question of the Universe of discourse, the presence of what Lacan calls the One-too-many (Un-en-trop) signifiers, which is also what is lacking, what is lacking in the signifying chain, in so far, very precisely, as there is no Universe of discourse. Too much and too little amount to the same thing, in this case. One too Many of the signifying chain as such is written as −1. Why is it −1 instead of a series of +1? Because the series of +1 seek to fill the gap left by the −1. The One too many is an example of discourse and covers over for −1 and a missing or lacking signifier and for this reason Lacan says that −1 is the symbol for an incomplete system that now in the current age substitutes for the Universe of a complete discourse.

The number 1 creates the symbolic system but −1 means it is incomplete. Because of the incompleteness, there are One-too-Many signifiers in the system. For the Imaginary One-too-Much means fantasy is always produced. For the Real, −1, One-too-Many means the Real cannot be signified within the Symbolic.

In order that any one of these letters whatsoever can take the place of all the others, it is necessary for one letter to be barred from it. For example, consider the letter Aleph (א) in the Hebrew language that is considered silent and as creating a space for the function of the "One too many" meanings among the signifiers. One too many is the constant sliding and failing attempt to generate the missing signifier/letter or Aleph. Lacan (2006) also uses the Aleph to represent the return of anxiety and the uncanny when the missing signifiers appear in the form of the uncanny in otherwise familiar territory (a◇$).

In addition, the figure of the internal eight serves to illustrate the solidarity of a goal-directed sentence and the retroactive effect of signification. The retroactive effect returns and goes over and repeats again the One of the circle or phallus, to reproduce the figure of the internal eight. The return, Lacan says, represents the uncountable that he calls the Un-en-plus (One more inside) or the Un-en-trop (One too much). This element does not pre-exist repetition and is an effect of repetition that Lacan calls "acephalic" or non-phallic that reproduces the phallic and/or establishes it as complement outside the phallic order. The anatomical genitals appear to complete each other and yet psychically the complement produces an excess that is not complementary to the relation between the sexes.

The One that is a zero is the same as the One of a cut that splits a surface, the border of which represents the One or O that is a zero. The phallus is a One that is One, unless it is missing, in which case, and in the case of femininity, typographically the One is a zero (0) that is an oval or ellipsis more than a circle. The internal eight is an O or circle with an oval or zero inside made by the cut that makes the internal eight possible. The zero inside represents the effect of retroactive repetition that as zero is uncountable or outside representation. The zero inside femininity that is uncountable and yet repeats the circle of the phallus "in you" more than "on you" appears in the uncanny or the Real of a hallucination. In this case the uncountable hole of femininity generates, for example, a tooth or an eye inside the hole to signify the imaginary phallus and the refusal of symbolic castration.

We said that the One too Many of the signifying chain as such is written as -1. This -1 is what appears missing under the bar in the "matheme" for the signifier of a lack in the Other. S(Ø) corresponds to nothing less than to the function of interpretation: to interpret what is missing in the Other.

Metaphor and interpretation operate by a signified or meaning effect. But this meaning effect (effet de signification) has to be specified at the level of its logical structure, in the technical sense of the term. The function of interpretation is a truth-effect (effet de verite) of jouissance upon the symptom. Language for Joyce was "L'elange" which as the end of English, or not being English, is the place where reading or writing English becomes a form of elation or jouissance (the truth-effect). This formulation represents the generalized function of the English language widely distributed upon the world.

Is there a being of the I outside a discursive or linguistic environment? The I of a fish and the I of a bird move in the environment without self-consciousness and at one with the air or water that moves with them. The same is true of the I of a child holding a parent's hand while walking. When the Je or the I of the signifier and the subject thinks, it is thinking within the linguistic environment, but also thinking with the body of jouissance or the heart of the signifier. The ego here is not thinking, and therefore is not. The subject derives its being from the "I of an Other" that thinks.

Thinking here means unconsciously thinking with signifiers without self-consciousness, but it also means that the I of the Other that thinks, refers to the objective forms of the world. True thought coincides with the form of the object. However, since there is no subjective Being in the Other for the human subject, because the Other here is an objective form of subjectivity, the subject has to find his/her being within the subject of the Real or what Lacan calls "the One's own non-being". Non-being or the negation of being refers to the negation of the ego, because in the Imaginary, the ego appears as an Imaginary One that needs to be transformed into the ego's own non-being, and the predominance of the signifier and the Real of jouissance over the ego.

Continuing with Lacan's seminar, the not-I, in the sense of the negation of the I of the signifier, is "What Freud brings us in the second step of his thinking called the 'second topography', as being the Id (ca)". The Id (ca in French, das es in German, or ben wo in Chinese) is something impersonal we approach in sentences organized around the passive or reflexive form of a verb that describes an action like "that shines", or "that is a shining", "a child is being beaten" or "it's raining, it's moving", etc. "It is not for nothing, that the very support of what is involved in the drive, namely, phantasy, should be able to be expressed as follows: Ein Kind ist geschlagen, a child is being beaten".

Because the I, as such, is precisely excluded from the fantasy, in the fantasy the subject is barred by the objet a as what the subject is missing. In Seminar VI, in his commentary on Hamlet, Lacan (1958–1959) argues that Hamlet wanted to know what kind of object he was for his mother's desire/lack. Hamlet wants to know what signifier is attached to this lack. Gertrude answers Hamlet's questions by talking about her qualities as a phallic object. Lacan places some words in Gertrude's mouth that refer to the demands of the drive, and Gertrude's demands for the imaginary phallus that follow from the signifier of a lack in the (m)Other. The words that Lacan places in Gertrude's mouth refer more to the upper signifying chain of the drive than to a normative response along the lines of how her son may or may not fulfill her social expectations as a mother. Gertrude does not have a signifier for Hamlet that he could use to define himself or tell him who he is (as an imaginary phallic object).

It is important to grasp that we have here the essential elements of what is involved in the unconscious. For everything that pertains to the unconscious is characterized by the element of surprise (Reik, 1948). The foundation of this surprise, as it appears at the level of every veritable interpretation, is nothing other than this dimension of the ego being not, or not-thinking, which is essential to preserve a revelatory character in this phenomenology. The signifier plays and wins before the subject can realize it.

The "I am not thinking" qua correlate of the Id (e.g., "I wasn't thinking, when I did something foolish") is joined to the "I am not", qua correlate of the unconscious subject, but in a way that they eclipse or hide one another. The ego eclipses the unconscious subject, and the unconscious signifier eclipses the ego. It is to the place of the "I am not" that the Id is going to come, the Id will come to the place of the unconscious signifying structure or to "what was thinking" despite the conscious ego. The ego will now say "I am that" which means "I am that object" or where the impersonal Id drive was, the personal ego shall be, which was Freud's formula for sublimation. However, Lacan interprets it differently. Instead of the Id of impulse becoming a civilized rational ego, the ego becomes senseless signifying thoughts but also, and, most importantly, in these senseless thoughts, the rational ego is not there.

We will now consider what happens to the I in the structure of masochism. Lacan made a link between the ideology of Sade and the imperative of Kant (Lacan, 1963). The subject should obey the ought of the drive, and of natural instinct, or, conversely, obey the imperative or duty of the moral law and not that of the drive, or obey moral duty instead of ethics being based on natural sentiments. The moral law dislodges the drive but lodges logic there in such a way that the drive is also logically organized as seen in the examples of sadism and masochism given above.

In the story of The Turn of the Screw, at the very beginning the girl and the boy were always described by the governess as kids of "fragrance of purity", "passion of tenderness", and "something divine". In describing the girl Flora, she said: "a creature so charming as to make it a great fortune to have to do with her. She was the most beautiful child I had ever seen" and the boy: "I have never found to the same degree in any child – his describable little air of knowing nothing in the world but love". We know with the development of the plot, this "sweetness of innocence" is conspired with the intention of not showing the sexual secret of the two ghosts. That's what makes the governess feel so horrified by it. The ought of the moral law is conspired to dislodge the drive, but, instead, the moral law is used to promote and organize the violations of the law. The pretension of innocence is an intentional mask for Quint's sexual abuse of Miles.

In the first occultation (temporary disappearance) of the ego – in the place of the "I am not" – the subject is where the ego does not think but rather the unconscious signifier thinks: "I think where I am not". What we have is the appearance of the unconscious signifier (S_1) instead of an ego representation for the objet a, as well as the truth of the structure discovered as an embedded signified within the body of the subject. In the same way, in a second form of occultation, a flaw or the absence of the objet a is revealed as a hole in Bedeutung (meaning), due to the incapacity of any meaning to cover what is involved in sex. The symbolic does not have the signifiers to represent what is fantasized about sex, and, therefore, sexuality can be described in the form of a ghost story. The first occultation is the occultation of the ego by the signifier as the truth of the structure. The second is the occultation of the objet a.

When the objet a appears in the structure, it appears as a hole in meaning where a phantasm or ghost could appear. Where the ego is missing from the structure, or is not, when the spectral image of the specular image or the ideal ego is missing from the structure, when the ego does not see that the subject is thinking, or cannot give its experience a comprehensible ego meaning, then there the unconscious fantasy will produce a spectral perception of a ghost.

In the story of "The Turn of the Screw", the governess's first encounter with the ghost happened directly after she fantasized meeting someone charming during her wanderings on the hill. "Someone would appear there at the turn of a path and would stand before me and smile and approve". And then with the appearance of the ghost of Quint, her "imagination had, in a flash, turned real". The governess had the desire to meet the master and to be loved by the master. But from the very beginning this road was blocked.

Desire is lost on the way and each time the missing or absent objet a returns, what appears is a specter rather than the object of fantasy. The specter is the substitution for the object of fantasy. Here the subject is thinking following the logic of fantasy. But the non-knowing ego has no idea about it. That is why the governess's first shock by the appearance of the spectra was quickly substituted by the second surprise of the wrong image: "My second was a violent perception of the mistake of my first: the man who met my eyes was not the person I had precipitately supposed". She said, "So I saw him as I see the letters I form on this page". This sentence is very indicative of how in Lacanian theory the visual field is structured by signifiers. As Lacan says in the Seminar on the Purloined Letter, Minister D may forget the letter as the gunshot appears outside the window, but the letter grasps him, nonetheless.

To define the Other as the locus of the word is to say that it's nothing other than the locus where an assertion is posited as veracious or true. That is to say, the Other becomes the field where material implication performs its function. To define the Other as the locus of the word is the same as saying that the Other has no other kind of existence than being the site and locus of the appeal to representational truth. But, since to posit a veracious truth is still to appeal to the Other in order to situate this truth, the Other re-emerges every time that I speak.

For otherwise, Freud tells us, it is absurd to see an image in a dream composed of a house on which there is a ship, or a person running with a comma in place of his head. After passing a fresh censorship, the Other re-emerges every time in the visual and auditory elements of the dream rather than in the consciously logical structure of the sentence, or the dream-thoughts that have been censored.

In this sense, the matheme for the lack in the Other [S(Ø)] means that we cannot consider our experience unless we start from the fact that the Other is marked with loss. There is always a signifier or a meaning missing in a dream (lack of a signifier).

From Lacanian theory we know that phylogenetically the first marks or unary traces appeared to represent and mark the death of an animal. Since ontogeny recapitulates phylogeny, meaning that the development of the individual recapitulates the development of the species, we find the first marks of symbolization not so much in Freud's "Fort Da" example that represents the presence and absence of the mother, but rather in the signifiers that mark what the mother desires in the father (that she lacks). This indeed, in effect, is what is involved, in the primal symbolic castration affecting the maternal being. The Other is marked with the mark of the unmarked or the mark of the loss. Lacan says we perceive it very quickly in tiny signs.

There is a loss of being for the ego: the subject speaks or thinks where the ego is not. This loss of the ego is the same loss that is experienced with the loss of the imaginary phallus or the objet a that a child is for their mother. When symbolization arises in the field of the Other, the imaginary ego and phallus are both lost. The castration or lack in the mother by the same movement is continued unto the subject. However, the loss involved in imaginary castration, when and if symbolized, produces a symbolic subject represented by the signifier. With the signifier more options are opened for the subject if the subject can trust the non-being involved in symbolization. On the one hand, the subject can travel with the signifier and acquire cultural and civilizing laws, and, on the other hand, the signifier also gives access to a different more objective yet personal signification of nature than that of primitive instinct or the imaginary. Daoism would be a good example of this.

"The Butterfly Dream" is the most famous story in the Zhuangzi (c. third century BCE), one of two foundational texts of Daoism, along with the Daodejing (I Ching): Once Zhuang Zhou dreamt he was a butterfly, a butterfly flitting and fluttering around, happy with himself and doing as he pleased. He didn't know he was Zhuang Zhou. Suddenly he woke up, and there he was, a solid and unmistakable Zhuang Zhou. But he didn't know if he was Zhuang Zhou, who had dreamed he was a butterfly or a butterfly dreaming he was Zhuang Zhou. He trusted and felt safe with his unknown being and non-knowing.

In the dream all characters are transformations of the I. The split Is have a relational connection with each other but the transformation itself becomes hidden, while Zhuang Zhou's dream is a dream of transformation itself. Whether Zhuang Zhou dreams of turning into a butterfly or a butterfly dreams of turning into Zhuang Zhou, here there is no difference between subject and object. There is no inside or outside. Rather, it is like the child's Fort-Da game, where presence and absence take an equal position.

The dream gives no place for the imaginary phallus or the ego, because in the dream, the subject is the dream itself. Both the dream and the subject are part of a network of signifiers. Zhuang Zhou and the butterfly become pure signifiers and the symbolic transformation is ultimately presented in a question form. Both Zhuang Zhou and everyone else coming across this question when reading Zhuang Zhou are fascinated by the state of "unknown-knowing" about Being.

When Zhuang Zhou dreamt he was a butterfly and woke up, he said to himself: "Soon I awaked, and there I was". He does not doubt for an instant being able to overcome this tiny problem of his identity of being Zhuang Zhou. He says to himself: "It is only a dream" (Soon I awaked, and there I was) and it is precisely in this that the dream lacks social external or objective reality. The conscious ego of Zhuang Zhou depends on the fact that the object is seen. Because we see the butterfly outside of ourselves, we don't think we can be the butterfly or that the butterfly cannot be Zhuang Zhou. This is what Lacan calls the traitorous aspect of the world of vision.

That the being of the butterfly, or the non-being of the ego, is here nothing other than what designates him/her for his part as Je or signifier represents an ascent to the signifier and symbolization of what originally was a biological or semiotic sign in the form of a stain in a shell or mollusk, at the level of the organism, of something which in evolution will become the eye of vision.

A stain in a shell represents what organizes the symbolic order as a −1 or something missing like a hole that sets the orbits of the signifying chain circling around the objet a that has gone missing. The signifier represents the subject in relationship to its missing objects.

The fact that there are signifiers missing in the Symbolic and that the Real itself cannot be said by language leads to the fact that truth within the Symbolic can only be half-said. That truth in the Symbolic can only be half-said means that there are different contested truths, and this in turn results in what Lacan calls the downfall of the Other. In the Symbolic there is always a number or letter missing, and therefore propositional statements can never say the truth of the Real of jouissance. This state of affairs leads to the downfall of the Other because, for example, in psychoanalysis so many contested truths about Freud's and Lacan's work have led to the downfall of psychoanalysis as a discipline.

The lack in the Other is a phenomenon, which is not to be considered as a happening due to a defect, but as a fact of structure, as the point of prudence with respect to speech and the word well said. The lack in the Other solicits us to advance in the most discerning way, with the most discrete steps, to designate the substantial point of the structure. This is to avoid the confusion of a renewed form of positivism in the sense of a complete and consistent form of objective knowledge. In contrast to a complete knowledge without lack, the lack in the Other is a moment of prudence and discernment leading to the apprehension and temporary vanishing of the structure.

The kernel of the unconscious is a thinking that is not in any way attributable to the ego of a subjective unit. Ucs. thinking is connected to an "I am not", clearly marked by the structure of the dream as the inmixing of subjects, namely, as the unfixable, indeterminate character of the subject assuming the thinking of the unconscious. All the characters in the dream represent the ego of the dreamer as another (the reverse of the process of identification where the other becomes the ego), while the subject is the dream itself. These two modes of the subject make the subject appear quite different in a dream.

If unconscious thinking is not attributable to ego, what about actions, are they also not attributable to the ego? Whether thinking and actions, and the thinking that is preparatory of action, are attributed to the unconscious subject, or they attributed to the conscious ego, in either case, the ego will be affected by the action. Unconscious thinking is orthogonal to the imaginary ego. The paradigm of this form of thinking is the dream, where different alter egos stand in for the ego of the subject. Alternative alter egos represent the ego because the ego has no inherent nature, and instead is represented by the signifier in language and by images of others in dreams. Lack of inherent nature is another way of speaking of what Lacan calls the unfixable, indeterminate character of the subject. The unfixable, undetermined aspect of the subject refers to the subject of and in the Real.

The singular subject of the Real and of jouissance is mediated by the function of metaphor that represents the subject of the signifier as a collectivity. For Lacan, reflex actions, motor discharge, or "non-reflective" movements, associated with instinctual actions, reproduction, and the Imaginary, are movements but not human actions proper. Instead, human actions are mediated by the signifier and signification. What does an act mean? An act is not the same as the manifestation of movement. An involuntary reflex is not an act. What is sought in the study of the intelligence of a higher animal, where a monkey sees, or has an instrumental insight into how to get a banana separated from the monkey by an obstacle, has absolutely nothing to do with an act, according to Lacan. Most of the movements performed by humans throughout the day have nothing to do with an act. But then how is an act to be defined?

The difference between animal movement and human action is symbolization but also the capacity of a subject to take responsibility for his/her actions. But does not responsibility require awareness or consciousness? Animals are living beings but do not have existence because they don't take responsibility for their actions. Human egos narcissistically advance themselves through their actions, but this is not yet responsibility. Responsibility requires two things: first, that subjects act according to principles of practical reason, and, second, that subjects prudently recognize, take responsibility for, and build on the slender and empty trace of jouissance and well-being associated with the word well said.

For Lacan the subject in the act is equivalent to its signifier. In the act, the subject is signified by the action, or there is an identity action between signifier and subject. The act, nonetheless, according to Lacan remains a line (razor's edge) with two sides. The act could have other signifieds in language that keep the subject nonetheless divided. But the act itself, or perhaps the analytical act more specifically, represents a cut in the line of signifiers, altering the surface as well as the background aspects of the psychical and signifying structure. The act itself is a cut. The act is a cut, and the cut is an act.

Finally, the writing of a literary ghost story is also an example of sublimation in that it elevates base, or condemned beliefs and practices, into the quality of an art form. To refer to inner subjective desires or objects of fantasy through an art form is a form of sublimation. Lacan defines sublimation as what elevates an object to the quality of das Ding. Das Ding or the thing as distinct from an object (sache in German) or even the inanimate is animated by the mother as the main archaic object of a subject's childhood desire. Something of the Real quality of das Ding is preserved at the same time that it is transformed into sublimation.

The subject is perfectly "thingly" (chosique) as a Real subject. However, in Lacan this also has a One significance with two sides. On one side, the subject becomes an impersonal thing in the drive or what we call the subject in the Real of sexual jouissance. Sexual jouissance here refers to the first fusional jouissance and the second phallic jouissance. The Third Jouissance we have defined as a jouissance of Lacan's second definition of the Real. On the other side, the subject is a "no-thing" or a subject-qua-nothing, or an empty subject of the Real. It is this aspect of the subject of the Real that is linked to sublimation. However, this is the truth of a different jouissance (jubilation) that requires the intervention of the Name of Father. In the Real of the sexual drive, the subject becomes a thing or objectified with the phallic object or fused with the Other. In pathological conditions the drive becomes a search for an impossible form of jouissance that ultimately proves to be destructive. This, Lacan says, is the worst kind of thing. The Freudian thing, or the repetition compulsion, precisely.

Sublimation refers to how "a repetition with a difference" transforms repetition into something therapeutic that produces subjective stability and a dimension of satisfaction within the drive, and the Real subject. Sublimation stops the repetition and replication of the imaginary objet a. However, sublimation does not stop the lack since at some point sublimation ends (sublimation is not a permanent state), but this does not stop sublimation from generating a presence of peace within the subject in so far as the word peace is contained within the German word that Freud used for satisfaction (Befriedigung).

However, sublimation also needs to be distinguished from defenses such as reaction formation since Freud said that sublimation does not involve repression. One thing is to pretend to be kind, as the other side of hate, and another thing is to experience a natural heartfelt kindness. For Lacan the mask of appearances is a form of the symptom. Here he defines the symptom as the significance of the discordances between the real and what it pretends to be (appearance). This is ideology. For Lacan ideology is a symptom because perception itself includes the distortions of vision produced by the Imaginary. Perception, for psychoanalysis, is the model of ideology, because it is a sieve with respect to reality. Everything in social reality exists in terms of ideologies. Philosophers have always constructed ideologies based on a first reflection misunderstood as perception.

In conclusion, what is the status of the fantasy then? The objet a appears in the place where the ego is not thinking and is rather affected by the symptom produced by the formula for the fantasy. The fantasy itself is contained within a grammatical structure and a signifying chain that contains the a. Psychical, or Oedipal and linguistic structure, and the function of analytical interpretation, produce the truth meaning of the phantasy that in turn produces a therapeutic truth-effect upon the symptom.

References

Chuang-Tzu (275 B.C.). *The Essential Chuang Tzu.* Translated and Edited by Sam Hamill & J. P. Seaton. Boston, MA: Shambhala, 1999.

Eliot, T. S. (1918). *The Complete Prose of T. S. Eliot: The Critical Edition: Apprentice Years, 1905–1918*, edited by R. Schuchard & J. Spears Brooker. Baltimore, MD, 2014.

Freud, S. A Child Is Being Beaten. In *The Complete Psychological Works of Sigmund Freud*. I. Smith (Trans.), 3641–3662.

Freud, S. (1915a). Instincts and Their Vicissitudes. *SE*, 14, 111–140.

Freud, S. (1915b). A Case of Paranoia Running Counter to the Psycho-Analytic Theory of the Disease. *GW*, X, 242; *SE*, XIV, 269.

Freud, S. (1916–1917). Introductory Lectures on Psychoanalysis. *GW*, XI, 386; *SE*, XVI, 371.

Freud, S. (1918). *From the History of an Infantile Neurosis*. The Standard Edition of the Complete Psychological Works of Sigmund Freud, Volume XVII (1917–1919): An Infantile Neurosis and Other Works, 1–124.

Freud. S. (1924). The Economic Problem of Masochism. In *The Complete Psychological Works of Sigmund Freud*. I. Smith (Trans.), Vol. XI.

James, H. (1898) The Turning of the Screw. Public Domain.

Lacan, J. (1958–1959). *Seminar VI, Desire and Its Interpretation*. B. Fink (Trans.). Cambridge: Polity Press, 2019.

Lacan, J. (1963). Kant with Sade. In *Ecrits*. B. Fink (Trans.). New York and London: W. W. Norton & Company, 2006.

Lacan, J. (2006). Ecrits. London: Norton and Norton.

Lacan, J. (1971–1972a). *...ou pire (Or Worse)*. Seminar XI. C. Gallagher (Trans.). Unpublished. www.lacaninireland.com. Accessed December 21st, 2020.

Lacan, J. (1971–1972b). *The Knowledge of the Psychoanalyst*. Seminar XIXa. C. Gallagher (Trans.). Unpublished. www.lacaninireland.com. Accessed December 21st, 2020.

Lacan, J. (1976–1977). *RSI*. C. Gallagher (Trans.). Unpublished. www.lacaninireland.com. Accessed December 21st, 2020.

Laplanche, J. & Pontalis, J. B. (1973). *The Language of Psychoanalysis*. London: Routledge, 2018

Laplanche, J. & Pontalis, J. B. (1988). *The Language of Psycho-analysis*. Karnac Books.

Moncayo, R. (2008). Evolving Lacanian Perspectives for Clinical Psychoanalysis. London: Karnac.

Reed, G. A. (1949). Another Turn on James 'The Turn of the Screw.' *American Literature*, 20(4), 413. Academic Search Complete. Web. 30 April 2013.

Reik, T. (1948). *Listening with the Third Ear*. New York: Pyramid Books.

Wilde, O. (1891). *The Decay of Lying*. London: Alma Classics, 2016.

Wilson, E. (1934). "The Ambiguity of Henry James." In *The Turn of the Screw: Authoritative Text, Contexts, Criticism*, edited by D. Esch & J. Warren, 170–173. 2nd ed. New York: Norton Critical Edition, 1999.

Chapter 6

Metaphor, the Censorship Bar, Metonymic Desire, and Nomination

To illustrate metaphor Lacan uses Victor Hugo's well-known verse, "His sheaf was neither miserly nor hateful..." (Sa gerbe n'était point avare ni haineuse), which he had already used to present metaphor in his seminar on psychoses. Lacan used this example again in his essay "The Instance of the Letter in the Unconscious" in Ecrits (2006, p. 412), where he gave the two formulas of metaphor and metonymy discussed below.

We begin with an excerpt from Victor Hugo's poem quoted by Lacan.

Boaz Asleep

Victor Hugo – 1802–1885

The man's mind, clear of untoward feeling,
clothed itself in candor. He wore clean robes.
His heaped granaries spilled over always
toward the poor, no less than public fountains.
Boaz did well by his workers and by kinsmen.
He was generous, and moderate. Women held him
worthier than younger men, for youth is handsome,
but to him in his old age came greatness.
An old man, nearing his first source, may find
the timelessness beyond times of trouble.
And though fire burned in young men's eyes,
to Ruth the eyes of Boaz shone clear light.

For Boaz the imaginary sheaf represents a sublated Symbolic form that clothes him in candor and clears his position as a subject with respect to the imaginary phallus that determines "untoward" feelings toward the other. Instead of the imaginary phallus what appears is magnanimity, timelessness, and the radiance of fecundity, as Lacan calls it.

Metaphor's creative spark does not spring forth from the juxtaposition of two images, that is, of two equally actualized signifiers. It flashes between two

DOI: 10.4324/9781003424574-6

> signifiers, one of which has replaced the other by taking the other's place in the signifying chain, the occulted signifier remaining present by virtue of its (metonymic) connection to the rest of the chain.
>
> (2006, p. 422)

"One word for another: this is the formula for metaphor, and if you are a poet, you will weave a necklace of metaphors with it" (magnanimity, fecundity, timelessness). Metaphorical effects are produced between the two signifiers rather than by the replacement itself. At the same time, the replacement is more like a movement. The replacement does not completely cancel the existence of the replaced signifier. Instead, with the work of metonymy, part of the occulted signifier remains in the chain and continues to haunt the other signifiers in the chain.

"In Hugo's verse, it is obvious that not the slightest light emanates from the assertion that a sheaf is neither miserly nor hateful" (idem). The part in this case represents the entire man, so that things that can be said about a man can be said about his part object and signifier. The replacement works with the assistance of the possessive pronoun "His" ("Sa" in the original French). "His" helps the metaphor to refer back to the person of Boaz himself, which makes the metaphor understandable.

We said in the second chapter that if the subject attempts to cling on to the signifier as a form of identity, then the imaginary identification with the imaginary phallic signifier will only fixate the subject to "miserliness and hatred". Our argument corresponds to Lacan's further comment on the replacement that happens in metaphor. He says:

> But once his sheaf has thus usurped his place, Booz cannot go back to it, the slender thread of the little "his" that attaches him to it being an additional obstacle thereto, because it binds this return with a title of ownership that would detain(keep) him in the heart of miserliness and hatred.
>
> (p. 422)

The use of the words "miserliness and hatred" produce the pun effect: on the one hand, they refer back to the specific poetic line analyzed above; on the other hand, they touch upon the truth disclosed by the psychoanalytic concept of the "imaginary phallus". What props up this function is that the two words miserliness and hatred refer to the human subject. If a kind of phallic narcissism or an identification with the imaginary phallus takes place, then a man becomes a "prick" or a "Dick" leading a miserable existence, while hated by men and women alike. The phallus is not a signifier of a privileged masculine object, but rather the signifier of a lack or something missing that supports and makes possible the metaphoric structure of language.

Dick or "mother's prick" is a name and metaphor for the phallus misrecognized as imaginary phallus. The phallus is the signifier of a lack of the imaginary phallus, while the symbolic phallus is a missing phallus and its symbol, Φ, Lacan says, appears in the place of the null set. The null set is a symbol composed of an empty parenthesis within which not even the signifier of the empty set appears ({ }) an actual set without component elements, not even zero. There is a lack of a signifier inside the null set, and the null set symbol itself represents the lack of a signifier within the symbolic, and in this sense, it is also the signifier of a lack. The only difference here is that the lack in this instance does not represent the absence of the imaginary phallus, but rather the fact that the Symbolic lacks the signifiers to represent the Real. Φ represents something missing rather than the presence of something.

In the example Lacan quoted, Boaz represents quite the opposite to a phallic narcissist. His asserted generosity is demonstrated by the magnanimity of his actions toward Ruth, and how his actions represent both the strength and plenty of both his sheafs and future progeny. Lacan says that the giver disappears with the gift, or the signifier replaces the subject, only for the subject to reemerge in speech once again.

The imaginary phallus that has been replaced by the sheaf, as an object of need and desire, and thanks to the humility and virtue of Boaz as a man, is transformed into a symbolic phallus that through symbolic castration becomes the guarantor of the generations. This is what Lacan calls the radiance of fecundity. The subject of the Real is not annihilated by the signifier/object "sheaf". Instead, by being represented by the symbolic signifier, Boaz, as a subject of jouissance, becomes even more activated in the symbolic chain. Now, Boaz's light of generosity and abundance shines over the symbolic line.

It is the abolition or replacement of the subject by the signifier that generates the poetic spark according to Lacan "The signifier is the instrument by which the missing signified expresses itself" (Seminar III, 1955–1966, p. 221). Paternity advances in the unconscious through mysterious signifying paths and through mythical life events such as observed in the Book of Ruth.

When Lacan says that Boaz sheaf was neither miserly nor hateful, the substitution of Boaz for his sheaves and his sheaves for Boaz functions as the "point de capiton" (quilting point) of the sentence. The line has both a metaphoric (sheaf for Boaz) and a metonymic reading (the sheaf being or not being miserly and hateful).

Lacan writes that he was

> Brought up with the Bible, I was stirred by what Victor Hugo had done with the story. To use a modern vulgarism, he had sexed it up. In the Bible, Ruth lies down near Boaz, and uncovers his feet. In the poem, Ruth comes to Boaz having uncovered her breasts.

In fact, the story of Boaz referred to by Victor Hugo comes from the Biblical book of Ruth. Boaz there is the ancestor of King David, and Ruth is a convert to Judaism. Lacan says that Boaz's sheaf was neither miserly nor hateful. Here Boaz has been substituted for his sheaves, as a phallic signifier, and his sheaves for Boaz. To understand the meaning of the sentence quoted by Lacan, an intertextuality (to use Kristeva's [1980] term) is in fact needed between Victor Hugo's poem and the Jewish Bible.

Boaz was a humble old man, who knew he was an old man by the time he met Ruth whose husband had died and left her vulnerable to care for herself without the protection of a husband. Boaz allows her to work in his field of sheafs and tells his male workers that she is to be left alone among the men and the sheafs.

Although Boaz was old and held a symbolic position with respect to the phallus in acceptance of the lack and the law, his manhood was neither miserly nor hateful to Ruth who became pregnant by him. In a way, this story is the opposite of the Biblical story of Joseph who was the first interpreter of dreams with whom Freud identified. At one point, where Boaz was humble, Joseph was arrogant and told his brothers about a dream he had where his sheaf was taller than those of all of his brothers. As a result of his arrogance and their envy, his brothers threw him into a pit and sold him into slavery.

Metaphor is situated at the precise point where signification is produced by canceling or substituting another negated meaning. Due to metaphor, the imaginary phallus can only reach the threshold of meaning as a missing symbolic phallus. Lacan also gives a different example of metaphor, "Love is a pebble laughing in the sun" (2006, p. 424). Here a pebble can be understood according to the "Lathouse" principle. A "lathouse" is the aspect of the objet a that can be extended to "animate" ordinary objects that may or may not have exchange value in the marketplace (Braunstein, 2012; Lacan, 1969–1970). The pebble is a transsubjective metaphor about love that goes beyond the Imaginary. This is an example of love in the Real without narcissistic altruism, meaning that the platitudes that people say about love in the Imaginary are narcissistic fantasies.

In addition, between nonmeaning and meaning arises the signifier and concept of the human spirit. By being tempted to reject the signifier spirit, for its origin in nonmeaning or emptiness, modern subjects defy and compromise their very destiny. Here we observe the movement of signifiers in two kinds of metaphors. One metaphoric chain goes from S_0 (emptiness) to S_1 (human spirit), and the second one goes from S_0 to S_1, but it ends up in S_2. This distinction parallels the distinction that George Orwell (1946) makes in his "Politics and the English Language".

At this point of Lacan's thinking, metaphor's two-stage mechanism is the very mechanism by which symptoms, in the analytic sense, are determined. In his later period the symptom becomes a form of inconvenient jouissance more than a metaphor. Between the enigmatic signifier of sexual trauma and the term it comes to replace/repress in a current signifying chain, a spark flies that fixes in a bodily symptom. The signification of the symptom by which the symptom may be dissolved is inaccessible to the conscious subject.

Both the formation of the symptom and the dissolution of the imaginary fantasy are inaccessible to the conscious subject. But in the "inaccessible" lies the possibility of a cure. Lacan's later work focuses in the jouissance that fixes upon the body as the key factor for the formation of symptoms. Lacan was led to something beyond metaphor and the Symbolic due to the limitations of interpretation as a curative factor. Thus, the symptom is the suffering of the subject and also the signifier the subject wants to hold in its grip. In analysis, where the dissolution of fantasy might happen, the symptom is transformed into a sinthome where the adhering imaginary ego has been displaced into the new signifying chain where new metaphors are produced (I think where I am not).

Substitution – the fact of grafting a signifier substituted for another signifier into the signifying chain – is the source and origin of all metaphoric meaning. In analysis, the source and origin of metaphor could refer to two different problems/signifiers, both of which need to be spoken about in the sessions.

Logically, a denominator represents the repressed in the same way that the bar is the bar of repression. A denominator is below the bar, pointing at the repressed signifier. When the subject takes the position of signification produced by metaphor, this means at the same time that the subject starts to seek its own truth in the metaphor, that is, to take the metaphorical meaning(s) as the real meaning about himself/herself. The barred subject as a signifier usurps the position of the s, producing the meaning effect.

$$\frac{S_1}{\$} = \frac{\$}{s}$$

The relations between the S_1 signifiers of the two barred \$s and the small s ground the function of metaphor. Replacement of S_1 for \$ and reappearance or the return of the repressed (\$ and its signification) are two key features of metaphor. S_1 is the signifier for the object that the subject has lost under the bar of repression (\$). The repressed signifier then reappears in the subject's speech $\left(\frac{\$}{s}\right)$. S_1 here can also represent the signifier that represents and replaces the subject. The subject remains divided between the signifier and what it fails to represent in the subject.

For the second formula for metaphor that Lacan produces, two signifiers are involved, with two positions of one of these signifiers, and a heterogeneous element, the fourth element s, or the signified effect, the one which is the result of the metaphor:

$$\frac{S}{S_1} = \frac{S_1}{s}$$

"The fact is that S in so far as it has come to replace S_1, becomes the factor of an S_1 which is what I call the metaphorical effect of meaning". S in this formula represents a signifier in a narrative that has come to replace a repressed signifier rather than the subject (as seen in the first formula). The S, in this case, actually represents an S_2 rather than an S_1 signifier. In the return of the repressed, the S_1 produces a substitute (s) as a signified effect. The repressed is only written at the point of its return. In the formula below S (1) continues the process of substitution from S to S′ to S (1), S (2), etc.

$$\frac{S}{S'} \quad \frac{S'}{s} \quad \frac{S(1)}{s}$$

The S in relation to S′ as the repressed represents the subject of the unconscious at the level of the symptom. The repressed returns in the form of the symptom as a substitutive meaning-effect. The third formula above is the symptom formula for metaphor. As we notice, the common element in the three formulas is the small s. It is the meaning-effect, the symptom, and the place where the subject comes to take its truth. This explains why the subject is trying to affiliate itself to the symptom: the subject thinks he is using language to express himself, but actually it is always the signifiers that reveal themselves to the subject. The subject is a raft drifting along the river of signifiers.

In addition, the unconscious is supposed to be constituted by the strange relation of the signifier to another signifier, and we are told that it is from there that language takes its orders: it is of the nature of each and every signifier not to be able in any case to signify itself. The signifier embodies the proposition that x is not a member of itself.

What repetition seeks to repeat is precisely what escapes, because of the very function of the mark. The mark is original in the function of repetition. Repetition takes place, because the mark is repeated, but for the mark to provoke the sought-for repetition, what the mark marks the first time is necessary (the unmarked) to establish the Symbolic structure. What has been effaced by the mark is what is sought in repetition. The mark cannot not be reduplicated, except by effacing the first mark.

For example, in Freud's Totem and Taboo, the totem becomes the mark and Name that effaces the killing of the dead father. But once the mark is replicated, the unmarked is effaced from the mark other than as a general background of absence required for symbolization. It is the original unmarked that provides the support for the mark to be replicated. It's the unmarked, or the absence of the object/signifier that has been left out, that motivates the repetitive signifying movement and provokes the power for symbolization.

At first the mark is the mark of what is effaced or remains unmarked. Then the mark becomes a unary system of marks independent from the unmarked. In every repetition there is something of the origin that is not repeated or that remains unmarked although it is included or "sublated" as the characteristic of the mark to represent things in their absence.

This radical lack, this first lack which flows from the very function of the counted as such, this additional lack that one cannot count, represents the logical function of the mark.

The entrance of the letter into language structures discourse at its most radical point of lack. The function of the missing letter is to allow the others to function, and thus in the case of The Purloined Letter the letter is in waiting for its claimant forever.

In the interpretation of dreams Freud (1900) addresses an objection made to symbolism and metaphor as non-scientific. It is objected that Freud proceeds in such a way that he always finds a signified which will provide a bridge between two meanings and with this fashion of organizing the bridges, he will always go from somewhere to somewhere else. Infinite metonymical displacements of meaning never arrive at an exact meaning. Everything will explain everything else. This is why the function of metaphor that has representational truth as its reference is needed to stop the infinite displacement of meaning associated with metonymy and the Imaginary. Metonymy instead, as described by Jakobson, is the putting together of signs along the axis of combination.

The deferral of desire, and for Lacan the impossibility of ever realizing one's desire for a certain kind of "other", is understood as metonymy, just as Brooks defines metonymy as a plot-sustaining détour or deferral of the end. This, too, one finds in desire in Lacan.

Metaphor, on the other hand, Lacan understands to be what he calls "the quilting" of the metonymic chain, the point de capiton or "quilting button" that suddenly holds together a sequence of disparate signifiers in such a way that a kind of substitution of signs, as opposed to a displacement of signs, can be accomplished. Thus, Lacan says that metaphor stands opposite to metonymy.

> If we say the main features of metaphor is replacement and reappearance, what we find in metonymy is detour and transformation, and if metaphor corresponds to the creatives power in poetry, metonymy designates a great place for those writers in history who values the metamorphosis of human desire as more important than anything else.
>
> (Lacan, 2006, p. 421)

"Thirty sails", for example, is a metonymy that defines a boat by one of its parts.

> The example shows that the connection between ship and sail is nowhere other than in the signifier, and that metonymy is based on the word-to-word nature of this connection.
>
> 13

> But what does man find in metonymy if it must be more than the power to skirt the obstacles of social censure? Doesn't this form, which gives oppressed truth its field, manifest a certain servitude that is inherent in its presentation?

Metonymy is involved not only in the question of searching for another signifier to avoid censure, but also in the search for a newer or different signifier, and in the way a subject may think about something else to repress an undesirable signifier. In metonymy, the connection between the two signifiers has a distinct feature. The important signifier moves onto an unimportant signifier found next to it. That is what servitude means in metonymical displacement. In this way the connection between the two signifiers is established upon a kind of defense but we know that the safety of defense does not lead to resolution of the conflict embedded between two signifiers. The transformation produced by repression will always show its aggressive claws in the chain of masochistic significations.

In the Ecrits, Lacan makes one of his important contributions to psychoanalysis when he equates metaphor and metonymy to condensation and displacement, two of the processes operating in the dream-work and in the unconscious in general. Lacan refers to condensation and displacement as the two aspects of the signifier's impact on the signified:

> Verdichtung (compression), "condensation," is the superimposed structure of signifiers in which metaphor finds its field; its name, condensing in itself the word Dichtung (poetry and seal) shows the mechanism's connaturality with poetry, to the extent that it envelops poetry's own properly traditional function.
>
> Verschiebung or "displacement" – this transfer of signification that metonymy displays is closer to the German term; it is presented, right from its first appearance in Freud's work, as the unconscious' best means by which to foil censorship.
>
> (p. 425)

Then Lacan asks What distinguishes these two mechanisms, which play a privileged role in the dream-work (Traumarbeit), from their homologous function in discourse?

In other words, these two processes also play a privileged role in discourse, albeit in a more limited manner, as Freud believed. In addition, these two aspects may function differently in the dream work depending on the conditions of representability and "staging". The dream is the "Other discourse" where the images both represent and conceal the signifying dream thoughts, and time-space sense is canceled. In addition, in dreams, there are fewer or no logical connectives as used in daily speech.

> Nothing, except a condition imposed upon the signifying material, called in German Riicksichtauf Darstellbarkeit which must be translated as "consideration of the means of staging" (the translation by "considerations of representability" being overly approximate here).
>
> Let us say, then, (that in) dreams the considerations of representability and staging are like a parlor game in which each person, in turn, is supposed to get the spectators to guess some well-known saying or variant of it solely by silent gestures.
>
> (p. 426)

Just like in dreams, the silent gestures are the images which need to be deciphered by the words of the dream thoughts. That is, in order to decipher the images, to know their meaning is never the point. Even a simple point of meaning cannot be reached until the whole structure and the specific weaving logic behind it are disclosed and realized. Until then, the scene unfolds before the eyes, but at the same time, there is still a stain or blind point in the scene that leads to infinite displacements. In another dimension, the blind spot also represents the enigmatic kernel of the dream, and an opening unto the Real, from which new names and signifiers may emerge that may put a stop to the infinite sliding of meaning.

> The rest of the dream revision is termed "secondary" by Freud, taking on its value from what is at stake: they are fantasies or daydreams, Tagtraum (day-dream), to use the term Freud prefers to use to situate them in their wish-fulfilling function (Wunscherfiillung – wish fulfillment). Given that these fantasies may remain unconscious, their distinctive feature is clearly their signification. Now, Freud tells us that their role in dreams is either to serve as signifying elements for the statement of the unconscious thought (Traumgedanke-dream thought), or to be used in the secondary revision that occurs – that is, in a function not to be distinguished, he says, from our waking thought (yon unserem wachen Denken nicht u unterscheideri- not different from our waking thinking).
>
> I have given the name of dream-work to the process which, with the co-operation of the censorship, converts the latent thoughts into the manifest content of the dream. It consists of a peculiar way of treating the preconscious material of thought, so that its components parts become condensed, its psychical emphasis becomes displaced, and the whole of it is translated into visual images or dramatized and completed by a deceptive secondary revision.
>
> This interpretive function is not peculiar to dreams. It is the same work of logical coordination which we carry out upon our sensations while we are awake. The mind endeavors to carry out upon these incoherent trains of hallucinations the same work of logical coordination that it carries out upon sensations during the daytime. It connects up all these detached images by an imaginary link and stops up any excessively wide gaps between them. p. 939. The interpretation of dreams.

Freud cites the example of Silberer who forced himself to transform thoughts into images by engaging in intellectual activities while in a state of fatigue and drowsiness. Thoughts were replaced by visions that are substitutes for abstract thoughts. Silberer wanted to simultaneously think the arguments of Kant and Schopenhauer on a particular topic, but he could not hold both arguments in his mind at the same time. Instead, when he tried to retrieve the arguments of Kant, the Kant memory "dossier" appeared as a concrete symbol or dream picture: "I was asking for information from a disobliging secretary who was bent over his writing table and refused to put himself out at my insistent demand. He half straitened himself and gave me a disagreeable and uncomplying look" (p. 941).

The intellectual function demands logical connections from mental material but due to censorship logical connections have been deleted from a dream. The secondary revision gets rid of disconnectedness and replaces it with a new fantasized meaning. If the dream work is not able to establish a true logical connection between dream thoughts, it does not hesitate to fabricate a false one. The dream thoughts are regressively transformed and worked over into a wishful phantasy. The dream thought and wish is hallucinated or regresses to hallucination. In dreams fantasies are perceived as in psychosis, rather than thought about as in neurosis. Although the fantasy can be said to be false or fiction, it can still lead to true conclusions based on the logical structure in which the fantasy is embedded.

Freud believes fantasies are inherent to dream formation. First, dream thoughts use fantasies to reveal themselves. As the dream thoughts become complicated, this task needs to be actualized through the process of substitution and displacement. That is to say, the dream thoughts go through a kind of "fantasization" under the workings of substitution and displacement. This transformation corresponds to the unconscious logic of the fantasy. The fantasy establishes a false logical connection between images, but this false premise can lead to true conclusions (material implication) once through association the dream image content is decoded back into logical dream thoughts.

Second, people are tempted to understand the dream content as they understand the ideas they have in conscious life. As Lacan says, "Given that these fantasies may remain unconscious, their distinctive feature is clearly their signification". This is why the analysis works upon the signification of the dream thoughts rather than the meaning or the signified in the dream because meaning in a dream is always the result of the first and secondary "fantasization". Signification is the hiding away of the dream thoughts by making fantasies real and waking daydreams the substance of life itself.

Lacan's main interest in metaphor and metonymy is to represent the topography of the unconscious. This topography is defined by the algorithm:

$$\frac{S}{s}$$

"What has permitted me to elaborate concerning the impact of the signifier on the signified allows for its transformation into":

$$f(S)\frac{1}{s},$$

"It is on the basis of the copresence in the signified not only of the elements of the horizontal signifying chain but also of its vertical dependencies, that I have demonstrated the effects, distributed in accordance with two fundamental structures, in metonymy and metaphor". The horizontal signifying chain refers to how with the S in the brackets as a function Lacan indicates that signifiers can always be replaced as variables. The vertical dependencies refer, in turn, to metaphoric substitutions of S or S_1 for s.

Thus, metonymy and metaphor can be represented by the following formula:

$$f(S \ldots S')S \cong S(—)$$

In this formula, the functions of displacement and metonymy (S…S) is approximately equal to the function of metaphor and censorship (the maintenance of the bar between signifier and signified), defined as the subtraction or loss of a signifier (−1). The S_1, as the signifier of a lack, haunts the substitution and produces the signified effect where one signifier replaces another signifier that has been "subtracted" according to what Moncayo and Romanowicz (2015) have called the formula for castration that results in the production of 1 as an imaginary number. Phi as the symbol for the symbolic function of castration subtracts the imaginary phallus: Phi–phi (1.618–0.618) = 1. So, the bar on the left refers to the substitution and replacement, and the bar on the right refers to the production of the meaning effect and the two different dimensions of the signifier and the signified. Finally, the implication here is that metaphor, in contrast to metonymy, may function according to imaginary numbers in the complex plane. Metaphor is associated with sublimation that is also found in the i axis of the complex plane as the capacity to sublate the negative values on the x axis of the Cartesian plane (See Moncayo, 2023).

In the first chapter we said that Lacan says that it is no longer tenable to consider that there is a Universe of discourse, for there is something lacking in the signifying chain. This flaw in the Universe of discourse is manifested in paradoxical riddles that at crucial points reveal an incomplete yet consistent system. The presence of what Lacan calls the One-too-many (Un-en-trop), which is also what is lacking in the signifying chain, in so far, very precisely, as there is no Universe of discourse. One too Many of the signifying chain as such is written as [S (—) s] or S-s. Why is it −1 instead of a series of +1? Because in metonymy the series of +1 (S … S′) seek to fill the gap left by the −1. The One too many is an example of discourse and covers over for −1 and a missing or lacking signifier and for this reason Lacan says that −1 is the symbol for an incomplete system that now in the current age substitutes for the Universe of a complete discourse.

From this point of view, and however counterintuitive, we argue that the one plus of displacement and metonymy, through which desire evades censorship, is equivalent to the missing signifier as a function of structural censorship or the Sense function in language.

(—) represents the bar of signification as well as the minus sign to represent the barred or subtracted signifier. In contrast to this we can understand metaphor as the form that sublates the original signifier despite the metaphoric replacement, while metonymy is what is lost forever in the displacement. Such continuing loss in metonymy gives birth to desire as stated in the next quote.

> that is, metonymic structure, indicating that it is the signifier-to-signifier connection that allows for the elision by which the signifier instates lack of being [le manque de Letre] in the object-relation, using signification's referral [renvoi] value to invest it with the desire aiming at the lack that it supports. The — sign placed in () manifests here the maintenance of the bar – which, in the first algorithm, denotes the irreducible nature of the resistance of signification as constituted in the relations between signifier and signified.
>
> (p. 429)

In other words, there cannot be a relation between two signifiers without a censorship bar. The bar is inherent in the movement of the symbolic line since the lack is what makes the symbolic order possible. The bar is what generates an incomplete system, as well as the signifier and signified as separate dimensions.

Now we turn to metaphoric structure:

$$f\left(\frac{S'}{S}\right)S = S(+)s$$

Metaphoric structure, indicating that it is in the substitution of signifier for signifier that a signification effect is produced that is poetic or creative. Instead of the bar of loss found in the formula for metonymy (−1), what we find in the formula for metaphor is that the bar has been crossed and a value has been added. The added value here differs from the value added by metonymy (S ... S′) that constitutes the presence of what Lacan calls the One-too-many (Un-en-trop), which is also what is lacking in the signifying chain. Metonymy always wants to find a variety of additional meanings between similar or related things. Metaphor instead stops the displacement or reiteration of meaning with a 1 that is not a "One-too-many". The 1, in this case, functions as an imaginary number (i) that is a concept that like a metaphor does not have literal existence and could be quite different from what it is replacing and interacting with.

Lacan's psychoanalytic use of metaphor and metonymy differs somewhat with the way these figures are used in language and literature. Within Lacanian theory metonymy refers more to the Imaginary, while metaphor is Symbolic. For example, contrast the advertisement used to sell a car that features a beautiful woman standing by the car versus the use of metaphor to represent a concept, a logic, or truth. In the first case, the car is a phallic or sexual signifier that conceals the sexual signifier at the same time, while the second sublates the imaginary phallic signifier into a higher or more abstract concept.

For example, think of the contrast between the Name of the Father as a dignified metaphor, and the vulgar image of the imaginary phallus that the metaphor also signifies. Other examples are represented by the Imagination and how signifiers are embedded in images and paintings. Magritte's paintings "The Pleasure Principle" and "The Therapist II" would be cases in point. The "no-head" or "no-chest" are respectively represented by the sky and the sun. In other words, an affirmative image is functioning as no or negation according to the context. There is a missing and expected ordinary piece whose place is occupied by It or das Ding.

Derrida (1975) also wonders whether the nakedness of meaning is covered over by the veiling forms of metaphor. He cites Condillac in "De l'art d'ecrire": "Metaphors are transparent veils that permit us to see what they cover, or the costumes beneath which we recognize the person masked" (p. 34). However, the metaphor of truth, or truth as metaphor, is not the truth of desire, but the truth represented by the sublation of desire. For example, Derrida says that nakedness does not belong to nature, and rather finds its truth in the social or spiritual value of modesty and moderation. Or think of Shakespeare describing Juliette with the metaphor of the sun. The naked truth is a signifying truth of desire, not the truth of jouissance as such outside the text. Is Juliette as the sun a signifier of sexual desire and phallic jouissance, or of a different form of jouissance? The objet a "reigns" over the subject through the sublated metaphor of the sun. The objects of desire circle around the void of absence (of the objet a), the same way planets circle around the sun.

Metaphor also represents how a figure of speech replaces another figure of speech, or how a first text is replaced by a second one. Is the truth revealed or feigned in fiction? Is the fiction true or is the truth fictional? Does the artistry of Poe reveal the truths of psychoanalysis in a disguised literary form, and/or does a psychoanalytic reading of the letter in terms of the phallus, as an imaginary object or a missing phallic signifier, reduce the false fictions of Poe to the scientific truths of psychoanalysis? Poe's text is also consistent with the Bible where to reveal nakedness refers to sexuality, the phallus, and the unveiling of castration.

When Lacan says that "love is a pebble laughing at the sun", metaphor here represents an artistic rather than a scientific concept. However, when a pebble's laugh functions as a non-sexual metaphor of love, a pebble, in this case, could also represent the feigned independence of the subject vis-à-vis the object or signifier that causes the loss of the object cause of desire. The pebble can be laughing "at" the sun or "with" the sun. Laughing with the sun opens the entire field of metaphor proper (sublation) as a fundamental principle of cultural organization.

The analysis and secondary revision of psychical material can also be deployed for theoretical and ideological/political reasons. The aesthetic value or beauty of a metaphor is not dependent on unveiling or unconcealing sexually determined material. The objet a can also represent something asexual and not only how sexuality impregnates non-sexual material. Just as metaphors can be used to represent sexual love, sexual objects, such as the breast, can also be used to represent non-sexual aims. It all depends whether the objet a is functioning as an Imaginary or Real object. The Imaginary here is sexual and represents an aspect of the life drive, while the Real is asexual and represents a constructive aspect of the death drive. Although phallic jouissance is obviously sexual, the Real is larger than the sexual. For what is "asexual", the Real objet a functions as privative of the sexual. Through the use of the symbolic signifier, the non-sexual a in the Real may replace the imaginary objet's a that is sexual in nature. The asexual a, as das Ding or emptiness, is experienced "without code" outside the signifying structure.

Metaphor not only sublates the object cause of desire to a higher truth because fiction as a genre contains a truth that makes fiction interesting for a reader. Derrida argues that fiction resents this ground or guarantee in truth, and that this resistance of fiction to truth also represents a resistance of literary fiction or the literary genre to the general law of psychoanalytic knowledge. However, imaginary fiction resists not only symbolic knowledge but also an experience of the Real of jouissance. Imaginary fiction relies on the Real of jouissance but the Real of jouissance, the "no-thing" as das Ding, cannot be reduced to imaginary fictions.

A letter could also be a letter from emptiness, and represent unspecified things such as an opaque tile, an ancient empty mirror, an empty envelope, or a blank transparent page. What writing or message is contained in such a message: a story, a forbidden desire, a demand, or request? What is going in that world? From which world is the letter? Although we do not have a writing, or we have a writing in the form of a flash of light, we receive hints, gestures, an index, a trace, stroke, a strike, or impact of Real jouissance outside the signifier. No code or scale can be used for something that has no code or scale in experience.

Lacan's later concept of the signifier as a semblance, on the one hand, represents the example of the imaginary impregnating, and being wrapped up or curled around the signifier. In ethology it refers to those useless objects or imaginary bodily signifiers (from the point of view of the survival of the individual) that are used to attract a mate of the opposite sex for purposes of reproduction. Think of plumage color or antennae that serve no other purpose for an animal. Here we also observe the function of material implication. Color or antennae may be false or useless as a premise for reproduction, but they, nonetheless, lead to true conclusions (mating).

On the other hand, the signifier as a semblance also represents the letter as a semblance of the objet a in the Real. The signifier is functioning as a semblance of the "ex-sistent" or inexistent unreal Real. The Real is unreal because it does not correspond to social reality. Social reality, in this case, is organized by S_1–S_2 relations, with S_2 representing a narrative or ideology. S_1–S_2 relations represent an intersection between the Symbolic and the Imaginary, while S_1–S_0 relations represent an intersection between the Symbolic and the Real. Here S_1, or a mathematical thought, has a link to the underlying body of reality, rather than simply being linked to other stories or social narratives.

Thought is involved in the use of the signifier in the structure of metaphor, while thinking is what is involved in the Imaginary, and the structure of metonymic displacement. Metaphor represents the repressive unconscious that filters and represents the drive and desire through the faculties of Sense, reason, and censorship, while metonymy represents the influence of repressed unconscious drives and wishes upon thinking and the logical structure of fantasy. The sign for the formula for metonymy is negative (—) because metonymy, in an attempt to eliminate the lack generated by the bar, simply keeps generating one-too-many-signifiers/objects all of which are also unable to represent or satisfy the drive. Too much meaning is the same as not enough signification or significance.

In metonymy and imaginary thinking, the signifier loses the positive (+) function of interrupting the displacements of the signifier, and instead the rapid proliferation of signifiers is driven by the attempt to avoid or close the lack (with imaginary thinking and wishing) instead of representing it. In metaphor the function of Sense, censorship, and signification adds, elevates, sublates, and stops the infinite sliding of meaning of the imaginary phallus.

> The + sign in () manifests here the crossing of the bar, —, and the constitutive value of this crossing for the emergence of signification. This crossing expresses the condition for the passage of the signifier into the signified, whose moment I pointed out above by provisionally conflating it with the place of the subject.
> (p. 516)

With the crossing of the bar and the emergence of signification, we also find Lacan's theory of the subject as a metaphor. "It is the function of the subject, thus introduced, on which we must now dwell since it lies at the crux of our problem". Here we find conjoined two aspects of Lacanian theory: the subject as a metaphor and the Name of the subject as a process of Nomination for the later Lacan. In addition, following from the formula for castration, the subject, metaphor, and the Name function as a 1 that is also a zero in the simple sense that imaginary numbers do not exist or represent inexistence functioning within existence.

> Is the place I occupy as subject of the signifier concentric or eccentric in relation to the place I occupy as subject of the signified? That is the question.
> (p. 430)

Metaphor's two-stage mechanism wherein one signifier is substituted for another, and the subject's substitutive representation by the signifier, produces two different kinds of results. First, when the signifier or subject is replaced or subsumed by a socially acceptable (the bar has been crossed) metaphor, then this metaphor and Name of the Father generate a denominating unconscious place for the subject as the signifier/signified of a lack. The signified imaginary phallus that they were for the mother prior to the symbolic Name becomes the signifier of a lack (of the object) that the Name represents for the subject.

The subject of metaphor lacks the imaginary phallus and also lacks any inherent substance as a subject of jouissance (Real). The NoF is an intervention on the drive that produces a natural underside: a first Real that becomes threatening to the signifier, and the signifier itself may also acquire sadistic characteristics. This is why a sublation of the drive and a new Name and knot of four becomes necessary. With Nomination the signifier of a lack becomes a letter from emptiness or nonmeaning to represent something of the subject of jouissance, or the "sujet sans substance" (l'esprit).

The subject, or perhaps it is better to say the ego, when identified with or adhered to the imaginary phallic signifier, is concentric or ego-syntonic with the subject of the signified as the imaginary phallus (phallic narcissism). Here the phallus as a lack, the unconscious, and the subject qua subject are ego-dystonic or eccentric to the ego. In addition, the lack of a signifier for the subject of jouissance is also eccentric to the conscious ego.

Nomination, as something linked to the Name beyond the function of metaphor, first appears in Lacan when speaking of the sinthome, and how Joyce came to make his Name to supplement for the deficiencies in his paternal metaphor. Lacan said that the function that Nomination and the sinthome played for Joyce was connatural with the best results that can be expected from psychoanalysis. In other words, in every analysis a new relationship to the subject's Name must be realized. In the knot of four, a psychotic must receive a new NoF through an act of Nomination. The neurotic receives a new signification for the NoF in the knot of three. The neurotic may also receive additional names without abandoning the NoF that for the psychotic did not mean much to begin with.

If the symptom is metaphorical, by contrast nomination does not work according to a pattern of substitution: it is not a replacement of anything else but sets itself up for and by itself at the site of reparation where a "slip" or failure has occurred. Metaphor remains within the order of the signifier, while Nomination works by means of the letter and the Real.

The function of Nomination is to set up a new Name at a Real place of jouissance where the reference or ground is the subject's body, rather than another signifier in language subject to metonymic displacement. When the function of the new Name is not in place, then the neurotic imaginary ego and alter ego can suffer from multiple personality and malevolent metonymic displacement. Nomination is what makes up for the fact that the subject is a "sujet sans substance" other than as a signifier or an image within a Symbolic system.

In the case of psychosis Nomination repairs the Imaginary's broken link to the Symbolic and the Real. In addition, the absence of a false hole or a repressed unconscious in psychosis is also repaired through Nomination and the sinthome that function as a new metaphor for the NoF in psychosis. Through the sinthome symbolic castration may be processed for the psychotic at the place where the NoF had failed.

In the case of neurosis Nomination functions as a way of rendering a new consistency for the subject devoid of the alienation associated with the patriarchal patronymic, the NoF, and the desire and demand of the Other. The new Name or new relation to the Name represents the Real unconscious or what about jouissance and the subject of the Real lies outside phallic signification in language.

The Name and not simply the signifier can be contrasted with the laws of nature. Nomination represents causality in the form of a gap, or the causal in the form of the acausal, as an arbitrary change produced by signification or significance (*signifiance* in the Real). Here nomination and the NoF originally associated with the Symbolic become something different operating between the Real and the Symbolic, which Lacan tries to represent through a mathematical topological structure. Nomination as the acausal or the absence of causality or a surprising form of chance is also suggestive of Tyche as an undetermined or acausal form of chance discussed in Chapter 1.

Nomination is a retying or renaming a new Borromean knot of four. Finally, the knot of four also requires transformations of jouissance as well as signification. When one form of jouissance is stopped another jouissance is generated or attained. Castration is an indication, pointer, index, or is at an early level of the signifier of the trace or traits to be exact (1 as the origin of numbers), of jouissance. Lacan's later work posits several types of jouissance and not all of them are malevolent. Phallic jouissance as the second jouissance stops the first jouissance of the Other and the third Other jouissance stops phallic jouissance by not being all under the phallic function of the signifier but still being under symbolic castration and the NoF emerging from the Real.

As already explained in Chapter 1, the Real here is a second Real different from the first Real in Lacan. It is from this second form of the Real in Lacan that the sinthome and the new Name emerge that will tie the Borromean knot of four. The fourth element is the second Real, the sinthome, as well as the new Name of the Father (the father of the Name) emerging from the second Real. With the first Real, it was the Symbolic that tied the inconvenient first Real and the Imaginary to the knot of three. The Symbolic fails for various reasons to keep the Real Symbolic and Imaginary (RSI) knot of three together.

The knot of three is unable to stop the repetition of automaton or unconscious determination. For the knot of four the Real is upgraded to the function of tying rather than breaking the knot and this required a new definition of the Real and new forms of jouissance. Convenient forms of jouissance, as jouissance value interacting with symbolic value, are what now structure the signifying chain within the Symbolic and enchant and inspire the human imagination.

As Nomination refers to the subject and the body of jouissance, metaphor refers to a mental process of symbolization. With metaphoric representation, the subject will find their own truth through symbolic thoughts that structure the order of language and representation. The subject is forever swinging between his/her imaginary ego-being (I think, therefore I am) and being a subject of discourse (I think where I am not). As Lacan says in the next paragraph, the question is not whether the signified corresponds to the signifier in my speaking, but whether the I at every moment of speech can be the I in the play of signifiers. When the subject takes the position of signification produced by metaphor, this means at the same time that the subject starts to seek its own truth in the metaphor, that is, to take the metaphorical meaning as the real meaning about himself/herself.

In the case of metaphor, the subject is represented by a metaphor that supports the function of the NoF and the place of the subject in the symbolic order. Boaz is represented by a sheaf and the sheaf represents him along with his generosity and fecundity in the lineage of generations. It is the sheaf that represents him rather than Boaz being identified with the sheaf as an imaginary phallus. At first Joseph identified with the imaginary phallus and suffered miserliness and hate as a fated consequence. The sheaf for Joseph was a metonymic signifier for his imaginary ego that he wanted to hold on to, while for Boaz the sheaf is a metaphor that represents and replaces him in the symbolic order. It is this replacement that generates the poetic sparks according to Lacan. In the vertical dimension, metaphor adds a signifier and is able to pass the bar of censorship or of the Sense function, because the subject and the ego vanish under it, or rather, come to be articulated by the poetry and treasury of the pure signifier. The signifier representing the subject in metaphor is the symbolic phallus as a missing signifier underwriting what remains unpronounceable within the metaphor as a form of jouissance.

"The point is not to know whether I speak of myself in a way that conforms to what I am, but rather to know whether, when I speak of myself, I am the same as the self of whom I speak." "Who I think I am is the 'cogito ergo sum' (I think, therefore, I am). When I speak of myself it is the signifier that speaks for me: I think where I am not."

And there is no reason not to bring in the term "thought" here. For Freud uses the term to designate the elements at stake in the unconscious, that is, in the signifying mechanisms I just pointed to there. The term thought here refers to the examples of the dream thoughts that signify the subject's desire and that are represented in the dream according to the conditions of representability. By using "thought" as the term designating the elements at stake in the unconscious, Freud differentiates it from conscious ideas produced in everyday life. For Frege (1892) thought has truth as its reference. In this instance, subjectivity can be objective and cannot be reduced to an imaginary form of conscious subjectivity represented by prejudice, pre-conceptions, wishful ideas/thinking, and an emotional/fantasized distortion of the world. Unconscious thought here represents how the symbolic structure as a logical operation structures the secondary revisions and wishful thinking associated with fantasy, daydreaming, and dreams.

At the same time, thought, or in this case a thought in the form of a naught of non-thinking, represents what is unsayable or unthinkable about jouissance and the Real. As Badiou (2009) said quoting Wittgenstein. "Everything that is at play, of course, depends on the line of demarcation traced between thought and non-thought, since it is Wittgenstein's strategic goal to subtract the real (what is higher, the mystical element) from thought". I would add to subtract thought from the Real of jouissance. With this formulation we arrive at three levels of thought and thinking: thought as jouissance or non-thinking (subject of the Real), thought as the logical and metaphorical articulation of the symbolic structure (the subject of the signifier), and imaginary metonymic thinking (ego ideal wishing and thinking), as already described.

Thought is beyond the grasp of the conscious subject but works to construct the subject of desire and the subject of jouissance. Seen from the perspective of the subject the mechanism of metaphor and metonymy is the mechanism of desire, while seen from the perspective of the symbolic order the mechanism of metaphor and metonymy is a mechanism of loss. And it is the loss mechanism that causes an eternal lack in the subject's desire.

When seen from the perspective of the Real, a loss, as a form of jouissance, becomes the emptiness that undergirds the symbolic order and the subject of the Third jouissance. Grammatical structure refers to the rules and principles used for constructing sentences in language. Rules and principles determine what forms are allowed or not allowed for constructing sentences in language. Metaphor and metonymy function within grammatical structure but are usually linked to motivation or what in psychoanalysis we call desire. Is the symbolic structure as a logical operation the same as the structure of language?

For Lacanian theory, the unconscious activity of desire is revealed through metaphor and metonymy. Signifiers of desire function as signified for a conscious series of signifiers which designates the position of the subject in language. Only the signifiers of desire, or the signifiers that represent the lack or absence of the object of desire, concern the unconscious with respect to the structure of language. Language rules and social laws governing kinship and sexual relations between the sexes are Preconscious and/or Unconscious in a descriptive sense.

The repressed unconscious contains repressed signifiers of desire that are revealed in the preconscious mind through metaphor and metonymy. The larger relation between linguistic and psychical structure is represented by the interlocking relation between signifiers of desire and signifiers organized by grammar rules in language. When we say that the unconscious mind is manifested in speech or language, we are not only referring to a relationship between unconscious desire, motivation, and the forms of language. The unconscious does not represent the "emotional" aspect of the mind but rather the relationship between repressed signifiers of desire and the general Preconscious structure of language in general.

It is very important to understand the function of Mind as something more than the primitive id, reptilian brain, or brain, period. Otherwise, with cognitivism or psycholinguistics, knowledge and cognition are reduced to techne, not as an art form but as a form of information processing controlled by the conscious ego and formal analytical reason (a form of rationality shared by humans and machines). What we don't understand is reduced to the irrationality of emotion, as if emotion was not controlled by mathematical structure.

> The fact that the signifying chain continues to unfold and continues to be organized in the Other, whether you know it or not, this is essentially Freud's discovery.
>
> (Lacan [1957–1958], p. 132)

> The small piece of Real enjoyment (S_1) that a subject can drain from the larger unconscious doing that escapes us, is what we call an act of wit (l'esprit).
>
> (Moncayo, 2017)

In this context, the unconscious structured as a language refers not only to the unconscious structure of language (in a Preconscious descriptive sense) but actually to the relations between the Unconscious structured by signifiers of desire (the reach of language into the unconscious structure of the drive and the reptilian brain) and the Preconscious structure of language. Metaphor and metonymy are the language forms that regulate (reveal and conceal) the manifestation of desire within speech and psychical structure.

Only the unconscious in a descriptive sense, or the Preconscious, is structurally related to the formal structure of language and how formal language obeys the rules of modern logic in a mathematical sense. In the conscious and Preconscious signifying chain, signifiers are woven together by metaphor. Metaphor represents things through relating dissimilar things: one thing is described by other things that share a main characteristic, and one form is used to describe another form (writing fingers for rays of the sun, early bird for people who get up early, etc.).

Metonymy replaces the name of one thing for another contiguous name commonly used for it: pen for sword, sail for boat, or greybeard for man, in the case of synecdoche as an example of metonymy. Substitution, as a rhetorical figure shared with repression, is common to both metaphor and metonymy, while contiguity is the criterion for metonymy.

Metaphors and metonymy are used to speak about material reality, but, more often than not, material reality is linked to the psychical reality of desire and its representations. Things are seen according to the intentions and desires of the beholder as the subjectively perceived world. Metaphor and metonymy in psychoanalysis refer to the signifiers of a repressed unconscious object, or a missing signifier, that functions as a hole or gap around which signifiers turn. Chains of signification (S_1–S_2) turn around a hole within which lies a repressed S_1 that is separated (due to repression) from the series circling around the gap. This is the false hole of Freud's repressed unconscious that Lacan articulates in Seminar XXIII. Obviously, this would have to be a case of an S_1 in a Preconscious chain linked to an S_2. However, because of primary repression, a preconscious S_1 is entangled with another S_1 lodged in the repressed unconscious.

To use the famous example that Leclaire (1966) gave at the Colloquium of Bonneval (1975), the preconscious signifier unicorn (from Lilly to "licorn" [unicorn]) and its associated meanings (S_1–S_2) is the substitute for the primarily repressed signifier of the imaginary phallus as a transitive signifier of desire circulating between mother, child, and imaginary father.

Within the language of jouissance or of the One (lalangue), significance is a function of the association between the phonological elements of speech or between the sounds of a word or signifier and the sounds of another word or signifier. Sounds function as a level of significance beneath words and grammatical structure. From the sounds of the world, and from the signs assigned to the objects in the world, to the sounds of letters and words used to represent a variety of things.

In lalangue, sounds do not convey linguistic meaning (like metaphor and metonymy do) and instead reveal desire directly through what could be called the mathematical structure of sound waves. Lalangue could be defined as the study of sound within speech and yet outside the system of language. Sound is related to desire through the voice that for Lacanian psychoanalysis constitutes a form of the objet a, cause of desire.

At first a child recognizes their mother's love and desire for them through the cooing sound of her voice more than the actual signifiers used. Sound constitutes the subject as an object of desire, and this refers to the pleasure experienced listening to the "the sound of music" that represents the desire of and for the mother (as in the classical Julie Andrews movie by the same name). Sound or phonology in lalangue is not concerned with the proper rules governing the pronunciation of words in language but rather with an equivocation in pronunciation, or sound "equivocality". Phonemes, as a sound of the voice, say more than the narrative content of statements in language. The sound of the voice (void) reveals what cannot be said in language or that is said in language in the form of negation: "It's not that" or "but not that".

The voice is outside the signifier but not unrelated to the signifier. The voice is Real while the signifier is Symbolic. However, when the unit is the letter, and the letter passes through the sound of the voice, the signified or meaning for the letter is in the Real of the voice rather than in another signifier. The voice in the phoneme represents the Real, or the intersection between the Real and the Symbolic. In Lacanian theory the voice cannot be reduced to the letter, and the letter cannot be reduced to the phallic signifier as Derrida tries to do in his critique of Lacan. The Real in the voice has significance beyond the phallic signifier.

Both the repressed Freudian unconscious and the Lacanian Real unconscious have the structure of a different kind of language – the language of the unconscious. The language of the unconscious here means two things. First, that repressed signifiers of unconscious desire function as signified for signifiers that, through metaphor and metonymy, are revealed in the Preconscious structure of language. Second, that in the language of the One or jouissance, S_1, as a sound in language, linked to the sound of another word, points to the sound of what is unsayable in the mother's desire with respect to the phallic signifier linked to the NoF. The language of the Other thrives on the metaphorical rather than grammatical or syntactic elements of language, while lalangue, as the language of the One or jouissance, thrives on the homophonic and phonological elements of language.

Herewith are presented two case vignettes as examples of the language of the Unconscious. The first will exemplify the homophonic element and the second the metaphoric, although in the example given, the two cannot be entirely separated.

An analysand, whom I will call J., had been struggling over not wanting to have "two sessions a week". He was also in conflict with seeing his struggle as having anything to do with the analyst. At the beginning of the next session, he made a comment regarding the waiting room saying: "your waiting room is 'too weak'". I have said that lalangue appears as a deviant or peculiar predication. Somebody could say, "This must be a grammatical mistake; no English speaker would say your waiting room is too weak!" And yet the fact remains that this was an educated native English speaker. The analyst, or the subject that is me but also an imaginary ego, responded by saying "two a week is too weak". Again, a deviant predication is matched by a peculiar interpretation. The two words week and weak construct a perfect example of alliteration. We know that in figures of speech, alliterations can also be recognized as a kind of metaphor. Here the fecundity of meaning comes from the condensation of the patient's repressed desire and a defense against the frequency of the treatment. This example also shows how Lacan emphasizes that metaphor is not effective because of the similarity between the two signifiers.

In this example, we observe that homophony is being used to challenge the "rules" of the treatment. The analysand represented here by the letter J. (the signifier is what represents the subject for another signifier – the analyst) and who was marked and effected/affected by being named after an aunt whom his father envied (the subject appears first in the Other) was caught in an imaginary ego-struggle with the analyst. To the resistance of his imaginary ego, two sessions a week represented an imaginary form of castration. I say imaginary, because he experienced two sessions a week as something being taken from him rather than given to him. Thus, he wanted to tell me in some way that it was not he but I that was weak. The analysand was making an imaginary or ego-defensive use of the symbolic link, whereas the analyst appeals to the aphanisis or disappearance of the imaginary ego and the appearance or epiphany of the metaphoric subject as an effect of the signifier. Once lalangue becomes linked to the Other via the act of interpretation, it is no longer a question of an imaginary ego-to-ego relationship. Now the signifier and the laws of the Symbolic represent the subject once again.

For the second example of lalangue, an analysand reports she is having sleeping problems because she is too excited thinking about presenting for a class. She continues with a dream where she is the teacher of younger students who come to pay her a social visit, and they decide to take a day trip. For the day trip, she will drive a big motorcycle, and the dream ends when one of the younger male students is telling her about his wishes and fears of success and expecting advice from her. She says she feels aroused by this. She explored the associative links between her thoughts before the dream and the thoughts/images in the dream itself. There is her love for a man teacher and her own desire to be a teacher and to be loved by male students. In discussing this and the difference between her thoughts and the dream, she confounded and equivocated the homophony between luck and lack. She sees male teachers that she loves as lucky and herself as "lacky", with lack being the main signifier of desire as a negative deficit state that diminishes her.

The beloved is lucky, and the lover is "lacky". A lackey is also someone in a subordinate position, and she would rather be the beloved instead of the lover. The Beloved is complete in her fantasy, and the lover is a "lacky" lackey. In this sense, in her unconscious, a man is a lover because he has the imaginary phallus, and a woman is the beloved who is the imaginary phallus that a man lacks. It is unclear when she is a beloved of her student whether she is beloved as a woman or as a man-teacher for her knowledge, whether she is beloved for what she is or what she has. She did not have a category or a signifier for a woman of knowledge. Although she wants to be desired for having an attractive feminine body, she also thinks critically of women who are very attractive and lack knowledge. She is also critical of men's "selfish" drive or desire to have sex with desirable women.

In the "metaphoric" example, an analysand is telling me how he has been able to be effortless and timely in his current university studies. He makes a joke on me, saying that he is dictating and that I should write down what he is saying. He associates this with being effortless in playing a wind instrument as a young boy until he had to put in effort to match the high notes of another student. Both of these comments served as introductions to his problem of not being able to put any effort into writing and finally finishing his dissertation. Then his associations go to his obsessive thoughts that his parents will die. He grew up in fear that his mother would die and says that his father wants to live forever but that he wants him to die. I interpreted that his efforts are geared toward remaining a child of his mother and not to grow up. If his parents die, then he has to be a man instead of his mother's boy.

Being a man for him means paying a price, such as losing his hair and not having feminine objects of desire. (In prior sessions, the analysand had spoken about his fears and desires to be a grown-up responsible man. He feared losing his hair like his father. He also had a dream where he was pregnant with a boy.) His response to my intervention was to quote a revered figure of his to the effect that being a man means having the baton of the phallus. "That's having something whereas for you being a man has represented not having hair like your father. Boldness is the baton", I said, and ended the session. Boldness is the baton that represents the symbolic phallus as a resisted absence that nevertheless generates a symbolic consistency and efficacy for the subject. What is being let go is the ego as the imaginary phallus of the mother's desire.

References

Badiou, A. (2009). *Wittgenstein's Antiphilosophy*. London and New York: Verso, 2011.

Braunstein, N. (2012). *El Inconsciente, la Tecnica y el Discurso Capitalista*. Mexico: Siglo XXI.

Leclaire, S. (1966). El Inconsciente, un estudio psicoanalitico. In *Colloquium de Bonneval*, edited by H. Ey. Siglo Veintiuno Editores, 1975.

Ey H. (Editor, 1966). El Coloquio de Bonneval. Mexico: Siglo Veintiuno, 1975

Frege, G. (1892). *Meaning and Reference*, edited by A. W. Moore. New York: Oxford University Press, 1992.

Freud, S. (1900). The Interpretation of Dreams. *SE*, 4–5.

Kristeva, J. (1980). *Desire in Language: A Semiotic Approach to Literature and Art*, 66. New York: Columbia University Press.

Lacan, J. (1955–1966). *The Psychoses. The Seminar of Jacques Lacan, Book III*. New York: Norton.

Lacan, J. (1957). The Instance of the Letter in the Unconscious or Reason since Freud. In *Ecrits*, 412. New York: Norton and Norton, 2006.

Lacan, J. (1969–1970). *The Other Side of Psychoanalysis: Seminar XVII*. New York: Norton, 2007.

Moncayo, R.& Romanowicz, M. (2015). Uncountable Numbers. London: karnac.

Moncayo, R. (2017). *Lalangue, Sinthome, Jouissance, and Nomination: A Reading Companion and Commentary on Lacan's Seminar XXIII*. London: Karnac.

Moncayo, R. (2023). The Trefoil of Jouissance. The Morphogenesis of the Brain in the Mind of Complex Numbers and the Subject in Analysis. Under Submission.

Orwell, G. (1946). *Politics and the English Language*. Oxford: Oxford Press, 2010.

Index

For Product Safety Concerns and Information please contact our EU
representative GPSR@taylorandfrancis.com
Taylor & Francis Verlag GmbH, Kaufingerstraße 24, 80331 München, Germany

www.ingramcontent.com/pod-product-compliance
Ingram Content Group UK Ltd.
Pitfield, Milton Keynes, MK11 3LW, UK
UKHW021723240926
475702UK00030BA/2388
9781032543758